YOUR KNEE REPLACEMENT

YOUR KNEE REPLACEMENT

A Patient's Guide To:

Understanding Knee Arthritis
Preparing for Surgery
Maximizing Your Outcome

Ryan C. Koonce, MD

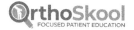

OrthoSkool
FOCUSED PATIENT EDUCATION

Cover design by David Litwin / Pure Fusion Media
Cover image © [Sebastian Kaulitzki] / Adobe Stock

ISBN: 978-1-7331358-0-1

Published in the United States of America

Why You Should Read This Book

A 2019 Google search for "knee replacement" yields more than 185 million results. Add to this the television, radio, magazine, and newspaper advertisements that promise a myriad of solutions for knee arthritis and consumers can be left confused. Which are legitimate? Knowing who to trust and how to navigate the medical system are significant challenges for healthcare consumers today. The problem is not lack of information, but rather, information and marketing overload.

As a surgeon who focuses on treating knee arthritis, for nearly a decade, I have been searching for a trusted, unbiased, and up-to-date source of patient education materials to help guide my patients through the journey of knee replacement. This book contains proven education and messaging backed by thousands of successful outcomes. It will help you, your family member, or your friend through this complex yet navigable process.

These are life-changing decisions: whether to have surgery at all, how to select your surgical team, how to prepare yourself and your home, and how to maximize your outcome. This book gives you the information straight – the good and the bad – so that you can make educated decisions about your knee pain. You will be armed with information that will allow you to speak the language of knee arthritis and understand your treatment options moving forward. If you are considering knee replacement, I invite you to start here.

Also by Ryan C. Koonce, MD:

YOUR HIP REPLACEMENT
A Patient Guide To:
Understanding Hip Arthritis
Preparing for Surgery
Maximizing Your Outcome

NON-SURGICAL TREATMENT OPTIONS
FOR KNEE OSTEOARTHRITIS

NON-SURGICAL TREATMENT OPTIONS
FOR HIP OSTEOARTHRITIS

———————————————

For online joint replacement education, check out:
www.OrthoSkool.com

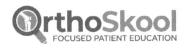

Contents

To Megan, whose endless devotion to our family inspires and permits me to pursue growth in all aspects of life. Thank you for filling my life with love and adventure.

Acknowledgments

Many thanks to the countless surgeons who patiently trained me in the science and art of orthopedic surgery. To the surgeons at the *University of Colorado*, who reinforced the critical concept of putting patients first, and later welcomed me home as a colleague. To the surgeons at *San Diego Sports Medicine and Arthroscopy Fellowship*, who showed me the joy in caring for active patients. To the surgeons at the renowned *Anderson Orthopaedic Clinic*, who humbled me with their knowledge, inspired me with their intellect, and shared their exceptional surgical techniques. Thank you doesn't cover it.

Lastly, thank you to the patients, past and future, who put their trust in me as their surgeon. It is an honor and a privilege to be part of your joint replacement journey.

Chapter One

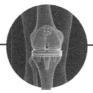

Introduction

I remember fondly a patient named "Susan" who told me, somewhat jokingly, that she had a recipe to "live forever" by keeping her body and mind active and healthy. At sixty-three, Susan still took her dog, Buddy, out for a morning walk daily, played tennis with friends on weekends, followed a strict diet, and chased after her four young grandchildren.

When she came to me, her right knee had already been hurting for six months. At first, she ignored the pain, thinking it would go away. She continued the healthy lifestyle that had always served her well. With time, the pain slowly worsened until it changed the way she lived. The more activity she engaged in, the more it hurt. She started skipping walks with Buddy and canceled tennis outings.

Although she was nearing retirement, Susan still worked full-time as a landscape architect and particularly enjoyed being outdoors and walking around job sites. Navigating uneven ground for work became nearly impossible due to pain. Time with her grandchildren was more often spent in a chair than actively playing with them. Susan realized that, over time, her energy, mood, ability to work, and overall health had diminished due to her knee pain.

Susan's diagnosis was "bone on bone arthritis" in her knee. We discussed surgery as an option. Surgery is a powerful word that can frighten even the bravest people. For some, it conjures thoughts such as, "invade my privacy" and "anything can go wrong".

Susan did not know how to respond. Six months ago, she was fine. What had started as an innocent pain had transcended to a diagnosis that was out of control. She was hesitant to talk about surgery and still had more questions than answers. She had always taken care of herself, so why did this happen?

Susan needed time to think and research her options. She talked to friends who offered a variety of opinions on what to do and who to see. She searched the Internet and found the information overwhelming. She then began noticing advertisements that promised quick fixes to relieve her knee pain. She tried some medications, supplements, an injection, acupuncture, and massage therapy; but nothing provided lasting relief. Eventually, she decided to move forward with surgery. As an orthopedic surgeon, I had seen many cases like Susan's. I knew instinctively that she needed a knee replacement, but I also understood that she needed time and information before proceeding.

Susan's case is not isolated. Many people with similar experiences don't know how to ask the right questions or get the right answers. Susan's story aligns with that of millions of Americans who have knee arthritis. Most are seeking not just information, but the right information about their condition and treatment options.

Finding the Right Information

Knee pain born out of arthritis, the leading cause of disability in the United States, can be like a tornado you did not see coming. It blows off your active lifestyle and transplants pieces of a sedentary stranger into you. Mild arthritis-related knee pain may prevent you from engaging in moderate to high-intensity activities. But severe pain may make it excruciating to perform even the most basic tasks such as standing, walking, and sleeping. Shockingly, your overall quality of life might be connected to a single painful joint.

Another surprising fact is that we physicians often do a poor job of providing trustworthy resources to our patients. The reason for this may be that it is not economically feasible for medical providers to sit down and educate patients one-on-one about the intricate details of knee replacement surgery. There is so much to cover on the topic that patients will need more than just a doctor's visit.

Have you ever found yourself asking "Dr. Google", as we refer to Internet medical advice, for information about a symptom you are experiencing? You are not alone. Millions of Americans turn to the Internet for help before making critical decisions about their health or the health of someone they love.

Unfortunately, searching for random information on the Internet can pose a risk to you as you may not know the right resources from which to make informed decisions. "Dr. Google" might be more of a foe than a friend. In addition to the Internet, you will find a variety of inaccurate media, outdated books, and seemingly knowledgeable family, friends, and professionals who are ready to offer their advice. You truly have to be careful about people or resources posing as subject-matter experts.

The ultimate goal of this book is to help you sort this information into a concise, accurate package that will help you make the best decisions. The advice you will read here is the culmination of nearly two decades of education, training, experience, and keen observation of patients being treated for knee pain. I have watched thousands of patients undergo non-operative and operative treatments for knee conditions, and I have witnessed their outcomes.

I have written this book for two types of patients:

1. Those who have knee pain and are wondering if knee replacement might be a solution for them.
2. Those who are in the process of planning a knee replacement procedure.

This book will help you decide if the procedure is right for you, and it will help pave the way to your best outcome.

Knee Replacement is Your Unique Journey

An instant fix, a microwavable solution, and a quick drive-through meal – these are the norms in our current culture. We want to press a button and let the machine give us an immediate answer. These days, we don't even have to press a button. We can just yell, "Hey, Alexa" or "Okay, Google" and these virtual assistants will get the job done.

When it comes to medicine, people are no different. We all want an instant fix to our health issues. We want a pill, injection, or procedure that resolves any health condition immediately. Unfortunately, there are only a few medical conditions where a quick fix is the answer, and knee arthritis is not one of them.

When this book talks about "knee replacement" it is not referring to a procedure, but rather, a process or a journey. And if you choose to embark on this journey, you will experience it differently than everyone else.

Imagine you have a friend who recalls a trip of a lifetime to Europe last year. He told you all about his trip, recommended which hotels and sites to visit or avoid, and how to find the best bangers and mash, croissants, and wiener schnitzel. You decide to pack up your suitcase and repeat your friend's magical trip. I can assure you, that even if your itinerary is identical on paper, your EXPERIENCE will be different. Knee replacement is like this. The human experience is a combination of personal history, our upbringing, DNA, emotions, sensations, expectations, and uncontrollable outside variables. The purpose of this book is to help optimize the parts you can control and understand the parts that you cannot.

How to Use This Book

This book is broken into sections based on patient needs. You only need to read as far as your personal journey takes you.

Chapters 1 – 3	For patients looking to understand knee arthritis and basics of non-operative treatment options.
Chapters 4 – 5	For patients who understand the information in Chapters 1–3 but are on the fence about moving forward with knee replacement surgery. These chapters explain the surgery itself, the risks, and the benefits.

Chapters 6 – 10   For those who understand the information in Chapters 1-5 and have decided that knee replacement is necessary.

This book contains some references. Feel free to ignore them. I've tried to reference only topics where the author or publisher deserves credit. Any topic for which I have not provided a reference should be considered my understanding of the subject based on my training, research, and successful experiences with patients.

   Learning about a medical condition and associated treatments is akin to learning a new language. For this reason, many medical terms are placed in *italics* and have definitions in the Glossary.

What This Book is Not

This book provides honest, efficient, and accurate information. Every surgeon has different training backgrounds, sources of information, and patient care experiences. I base the information on what most joint replacement surgeons would agree with. This book represents information that I recommend other surgeons follow in their practice, but your own surgeon may have different preferences.

   This book will not address the complex issue of pain in existing knee replacements or provide in-depth coverage of complications associated with knee replacements. If you have already had a knee replacement and are looking for solutions for ongoing pain or other problems, please consult a local joint replacement surgeon.

Conflicts of Interest

The author and publisher of this book have no conflicts of interest or paid relationships with medical device companies, drug companies, or any other financial incentives that would cause us to recommend specific surgical and non-surgical treatment options. Any potential conflicts of interest that might arise after the publication date of this book will be disclosed on www.orthoskool.com.

Chapter 1 Review

- There is a lot of information out there. Obtaining the right information is critical to understanding knee pain, arthritis, and treatment options.

- Knee replacement is not a single procedure, it's a journey.

- Everyone experiences knee pain and knee replacement surgery differently.

- Preparation and education will enhance your experience and your outcome, whether you have knee replacement or choose a non-operative treatment.

Chapter Two

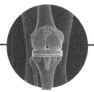

Understanding Knee Arthritis

The Burdensome Knee

If you have *chronic* knee pain, you probably remember a time when you were pain-free. As children and teenagers, most of us were active and not limited by joint pain. Some describe the feeling of their youth as "being invincible". We could run, jump, skip, pivot, and dance for hours without pain. Our knees were no different than our earlobes in that that it was a body part and not a pain generator. If you currently have knee arthritis and are considering knee replacement, your previously invincible knee has become a burden that you are acutely aware of every day.

In this chapter, I define the normal anatomy of the knee and the condition of arthritis. I also describe how the invincible knee can become the burdensome knee. With these building blocks in place, we will have the background to discuss treatment options in upcoming chapters.

Knee Anatomy – The Invincible Knee Before Arthritis

We are going to stick to the basics, but first, you should learn about the anatomy of the normal knee before we move on to what can go wrong.

The knee is medically known as a *hinge joint*: a joint that primarily bends and straightens in one plane of motion. The knee joint consists of **three bones** which play important roles in its form and function (Figure 2-1). The *fibula* is a close-by fourth bone that supports the knee joint, the lower leg, and the ankle joint, but does not play a key role in knee arthritis.

The three major bones are:

1. *Femur*: Your thigh bone. The longest bone in the body, extending from your hip joint to your knee joint

2. *Tibia*: Your shin bone, which extends from the knee to the ankle.

3. *Patella*: Your kneecap. This bone glides up and down in a groove on the femur bone as your knee bends and straightens.

The normal knee has two types of *cartilage* in it (Figure 2-1). *Cartilage* is typically soft and protects bones from rubbing together. All joints have cartilage in them. The types of cartilage in the knee include:

1. *Articular cartilage* (also called surface cartilage): This is a very smooth, slick surface that covers the end of the femur, tibia, and backside of the patella. Think of this as a coating over the bones that is typically < 3 mm thick. In a healthy knee, articular cartilage allows the joint surfaces to glide past each other with minimal friction.

2. *Meniscus* (pleural = *menisci)*: These are two c-shaped cartilage wedges that serve as shock absorbers in the knee joint. They protect the articular cartilage as well as the underlying bone from damage.

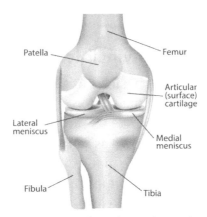

Figure 2-1: Bones and cartilage that make up the knee joint.

The bones that make up the knee joint are held together by soft tissues. Your knee has several soft (but strong) tissue structures that serve two purposes: to support your knee, and to assist with bending/straightening. *Ligaments* connect two bones together. They are *static* supporting structures because they stay in one place and resist stretching and movement. *Tendons* connect muscles to bone. We call them *dynamic* supporting structures because the muscles contract to apply tension around the joints. The ligaments and tendons within the knee joint are shown in Figure 2-2.

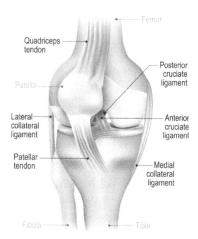

Figure 2-2: Supporting soft tissue structures in the knee joint include ligaments and tendons.

There are three *compartments* in the knee. Compartments are areas of the knee where cartilage covering two bones *articulate* (the medical term for "rub together"). There are three distinct parts of the knee where cartilage-covered bones articulate:

1. <u>Medial compartment</u>: *medial* means "toward the midline of the body", this compartment is found in the inner side of the knee.

2. <u>Lateral compartment</u>: *lateral* means "away from the midline of the body;" this compartment is found in the outer part of the knee

3. <u>Patellofemoral compartment</u>: this is the compartment where the *patella* glides up and down a groove in the femur called the

trochlea. There is cartilage both on the back side of the *patella* and in the *trochlea.*

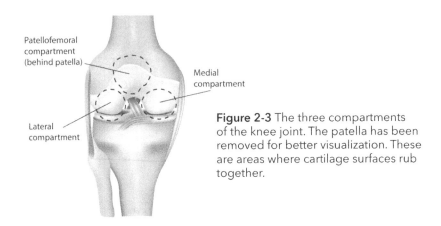

Patellofemoral compartment (behind patella)

Medial compartment

Lateral compartment

Figure 2-3 The three compartments of the knee joint. The patella has been removed for better visualization. These are areas where cartilage surfaces rub together.

Knee Arthritis – The Burdensome Knee

The word "arthritis" originates from two Greek words – *arthron*, meaning "joint" and *itis*, a medical suffix attached to any medical condition characterized by inflammation. When you combine these two words, you get a new word, *arthr-itis*, or "inflamed joint". Similar examples include *col-itis* (inflamed colon) and *bronch-itis* (inflamed bronchi).

Inflammation of the knee joint is often associated with cartilage wear. Cartilage wear has become synonymous with arthritis. Cartilage wear occurs when the few millimeters of cartilage covering the ends of the bone deteriorates, exposing the bone underneath. When a person has significant inflammation and cartilage wear, pain is the common result. Figure 2-4 compares the normal knee to the arthritic knee.

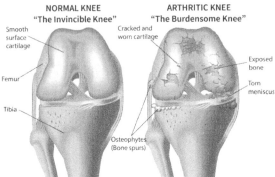

NORMAL KNEE
"The Invincible Knee"

ARTHRITIC KNEE
"The Burdensome Knee"

Smooth surface cartilage

Cracked and worn cartilage

Exposed bone

Femur

Torn meniscus

Tibia

Osteophytes (Bone spurs)

Figure 2-4: The normal knee versus the arthritic knee.

How Arthritis is Diagnosed

The definitive test to diagnose arthritis is x-ray. Physicians use several criteria to diagnose arthritis with x-ray, but the two most common are:

1. _Cartilage space narrowing_: Bone always shows up on an x-ray and cartilage does not – it is transparent on x-ray. A classic x-ray sign of cartilage wear is a narrowing of the transparent space where the cartilage used to be.

2. _Osteophytes_: As a protective mechanism during cartilage wear, outcroppings of bone and/or cartilage form at the edge of the knee joint. These are commonly called "bone spurs." Bone spurs are another telltale x-ray sign of cartilage wear.

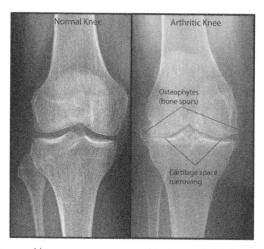

Figure 2-5: A normal knee x-ray compared to the arthritic knee x-ray. Note the cartilage space narrowing and osteophytes in the arthritic knee.

Using x-ray, your doctor can rate the severity of your arthritis.

- If you have _mild arthritis_, you will have minimal cartilage space narrowing.

- If you have _moderate arthritis_, at least 50 percent of your available cartilage space will be gone while some osteophytes may be present.

- If you have *severe arthritis*, in at least one area of your knee, there will be full-thickness loss of cartilage, a condition known as *bone-on-bone arthritis*.

It is important to note that advanced imaging such as CT scan and MRI are typically not needed if arthritis is seen on x-ray. These advanced studies are only helpful if the diagnosis is in doubt after the x-ray.

Common Misconceptions about Arthritis

Some people think arthritis is a material that forms in the knee. Arthritis is a medical condition, not a substance. You cannot scrape away, remove, or clean out inflammation and cartilage wear. It is less like the tartar that builds up on your teeth than it is like the wear on your car tires in areas where the tread is gone.

Perhaps the confusion is because when we look at an x-ray, we can see those bone spurs (osteophytes) that form in response to arthritis. However, you should know that these bone spurs are just a feature or sign of arthritis and not the arthritis itself. Removal of this feature does not cure the disease.

Regarding arthritis features, let us quickly identify some other features that often present with arthritis (although not always). One feature is *pain*. Arthritis-related pain is complicated. For reasons that the medical community does not fully understand, arthritis does not always result in knee pain. In addition, the severity of arthritis as seen on an x-ray is not directly proportional to the amount of pain you may experience. In other words, we cannot tell how much pain you are having just by looking at your x-ray. Some patients with mild arthritis may have severe pain, while others with severe arthritis may not have pain at all.

Another optional arthritis feature is *deformity*. In orthopedic terms, *deformity* simply means angulation of the joint. Some patients with knee arthritis may become bow-legged (*varus* deformity). This occurs when the cartilage on the *medial* compartment wears out faster than the lateral compartment. Other patients may become knock-kneed (*valgus* deformity), where the lateral compartment wears out first.

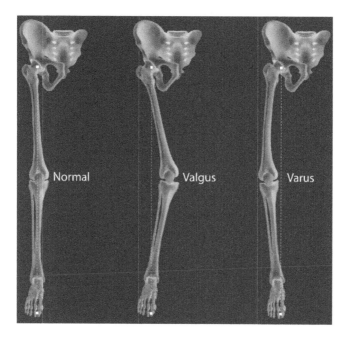

Figure 2-6: Normal knee alignment, valgus (knock-kneed), and varus (bow-legged) deformities of the knee.

Types of Knee Arthritis

There are three major types of knee arthritis. Each type has a unique underlying cause but produces a similar painful condition.

Osteoarthritis

The first is *osteoarthritis*. This is by far the most common type. It is called "wear and tear" arthritis because it often has no identifiable cause and is more prevalent with age. *Osteoarthritis* is commonly confused with *osteoporosis*; however, they are not the same. *Osteoporosis* is a problem within the structure of a bone that results in decreased bone density, which then causes bones to fracture easily.

Inflammatory arthritis

Inflammatory arthritis describes a group of diseases where excess inflammation occurs in the joints for unknown reasons, and cartilage wear follows.

Rheumatoid arthritis is the most common type of inflammatory arthritis. This is an *autoimmune* disorder, where the body's immune system is overactive and works against joint surfaces to break down otherwise healthy cartilage and bone.

Most people with inflammatory arthritis have seen a rheumatologist and are on special medications to treat their systemic condition.

Post-traumatic arthritis

The third is *post-traumatic arthritis*. This occurs when a trauma such as a fracture occurs within the joint surface leading to permanent damage. When the cartilage sustains significant damage, it may do well for a period; however, over the course of months or years, worsening arthritis develops.

What Causes Osteoarthritis?

This question comes up frequently. It is easier to understand why cartilage wear occurs with inflammatory and post-traumatic arthritis. However, osteoarthritis is complex and *multifactorial*, which means that there are several factors that contribute to it. There are *inherent* (things you can't change) and *modifiable* (things you can change) risk factors for the development of osteoarthritis (Table 2-1):

Table 2-1: Inherent and modifiable risk factors for osteoarthritis

Inherent Risk Factors	Modifiable
Genetic makeup	Excess body mass
Gender	Sport/occupation stresses
Age	
Minor injury	
Luck	

Inherent Risk Factors – things you cannot change

- <u>Genetic makeup</u>: Your genes play a large role in osteoarthritis, but their exact role is not fully understood. It is not as simple as skin color or height, which can often be predicted based on your parents. Multiple genes play a role, and the interactions and expression of those genes are under current investigation.

- <u>Gender</u>: Osteoarthritis is more common and more severe in women than men.

- <u>Age</u>: There is a clear correlation with age and prevalence of osteoarthritis.

- <u>Injury</u>: When a patient has a prior major injury such as a fracture within the knee joint or a ligament injury, we classify subsequent arthritis as post-traumatic. Patients may not recall a time long ago when they had a minor twisting injury to their knee that hurt for a few days and resolved without ever seeing a doctor. We believe that some of these seemingly minor injuries can result in osteoarthritis much later in life.

- <u>Luck</u>: Because there are so many potential causes of osteoarthritis and much of this we still do not understand, we tell patients that there is some luck involved.

Modifiable Risk Factors – things you can change

- <u>Excess body mass</u>: Excess body weight can be a sensitive subject, but it is clearly linked to osteoarthritis. Obesity has reached pandemic status worldwide. Body mass affects knee arthritis in two ways. The first is intuitive: increased weight (or load) on cartilage surfaces increases the rate of wear. The second is less intuitive (and maybe more important): excess fat tissue secretes molecules in the body that increase inflammation and are thought to cause cartilage surfaces to break down. When these two mechanisms are working together, they cause the cartilage in your knees to wear at a rate higher than they would if you were at your ideal body weight. See "Calculation of Body Mass Index" below to figure out your ideal body weight.

- Sport and occupation stress: It may seem intuitive that more weight-bearing activities and stress on the knee joint would cause more wear. This is the common historical teaching of medical providers. Research has not proven this to be definitively true. Running, for example, is considered one of the biggest stressors on the knee joint, yet several studies have shown that runners do not have an increased risk of knee arthritis. There is also a theory that exercise strengthens bones and joints and therefore provides a protective effect against cartilage wear, which may counteract wear. Here is what I tell my patients: avoid running, sports, and activities that cause knee pain because if it's causing pain, it's probably causing damage; but if you can run marathons without pain in your knees, it's probably fine to continue.

Calculation of Body Mass Index

Search the Internet for "body mass index calculator." Several will come up, and any will do the job. Enter your height and weight when prompted. Calculate your *body mass index* (BMI). Once you have calculated this, compare your BMI to the numbers below as published by the Centers for Disease Control:

Underweight <18.5
Healthy Range 18.5 – 24.9
Overweight 25.0 – 29.9
Obese ≥30.0

Obese Class I: 30 – 34.9
Obese Class II: 35 – 39.9
Obese Class III: ≥40 (also called "extreme" or "severe" obesity)

If your BMI is >30, you should strongly consider weight loss. If your BMI is >35, then you have a serious health condition that needs immediate attention. If your BMI is over forty, you should not be considering any elective surgical procedure until you have lost weight. This is a general guideline and may not apply to muscular individuals who are lean.

The Progression of Knee Osteoarthritis

The natural history of knee arthritis, regardless of the type or cause, involves progression over time. Symptoms include pain and inflammation. In addition, the inability to exercise and walk long distances tends to worsen. The progression of knee osteoarthritis is often in a variable stepwise fashion, meaning it does not increase at a constant rate, but gets better, then worse, then better, then worse, etc.

Figure 2-7 shows an example of the stepwise progression of pain over time. Note the areas labeled "*flare*". It is common for patients to show up at a doctor's office with a bout of severe pain in a knee that has been only mildly symptomatic in the past, only to find that x-rays show the *chronic* condition of arthritis may have been there for months or years. The period of flare tends to last days or weeks, but usually improves, especially after utilizing some of the treatments listed in Chapter 3.

X-rays also tend to worsen with time. Progressive cartilage space narrowing is the most common finding on an x-ray, and we will often see enlarging osteophytes and increasing deformity (more varus or valgus deformity).

The condition of arthritis encompasses a spectrum of symptoms where some patients may not be able to run but can perform all other activities pain-free. Another patient may have trouble standing, walking, or sleeping at night. On the severe end, symptoms can be debilitating and require a walker or wheelchair.

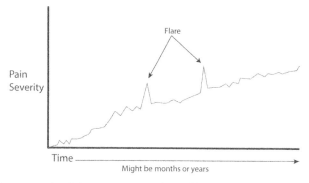

Figure 2-7: An example of the stepwise and variable progression of arthritis symptoms over time. The severity of pain over time will be different for every knee. Note the areas of worsening and improvement, with severe worsening known as "flare".

Chapter 2 Review

- Arthritis = joint inflammation + cartilage wear.

- Arthritis is not a substance in your knee, it is a condition.

- Bone spurs are a result of arthritis and a sign we see on x-ray. They are not the cause of pain and are not the underlying problem.

- There are three main types of arthritis:

  1. Osteoarthritis
  2. Inflammatory arthritis
  3. Post-traumatic arthritis

- The cause of osteoarthritis is *multifactorial*, with many factors that you cannot control.

- Body mass index is important in determining your risk for arthritis and your risk for overall health problems.

- Arthritis tends to progress over time with respect to symptoms and x-ray findings, respectively.

- A "flare" of arthritis is a dramatic acute worsening of symptoms that lasts from days to weeks but usually improves.

- Arthritis encompasses a spectrum of diseases; symptoms can range from very mild discomfort to severe and debilitating pain.

Chapter Three

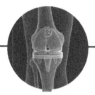

Alternatives to Knee Replacement Surgery

The Kitchen Sink

You've seen a medical provider, had an examination and x-rays, and been told that you have knee arthritis. Now what? This chapter introduces an important concept that must be clearly communicated.

If you have moderate or severe knee arthritis that is responsible for daily pain, we do not have the technology to give you your previously "invincible knee" back. Anyone who promises otherwise is not giving you accurate information. Most people with severe arthritis aren't looking for this; they just want to be active without daily pain. Living an active life is most definitely achievable if you have been diagnosed with knee arthritis. The answer likely lies in this or the following chapter.

> **Important Note:** This chapter describes non-operative treatments relevant to knee *osteoarthritis* and *post-traumatic arthritis*. Inflammatory arthritis has different treatment options that should be discussed with your primary care provider or rheumatologist.

The Kitchen Sink

I am a strong proponent of exhausting all non-operative options prior to taking on major surgery. When you avoid surgery you also avoid all the risks that come with it. Knee replacement is major surgery and has risks that will be covered in Chapter 4.

But first, let's talk about potentially avoiding surgery by throwing the proverbial kitchen sink at the knee. In this chapter, we will outline what I consider to be the first, second, and third-line treatment options and include a brief discussion. For a more in-depth discussion of each treatment, please check out the companion book *Non-Surgical Treatment Options for Knee Osteoarthritis, 2019 Edition.*

Non-Operative Alternatives to Knee Replacement

Once the cartilage is worn away from the knee joint, we currently do not have a reliable method to put this cartilage back or replace the worn surfaces without surgery. Let's be clear on this: currently, there are no available injections, supplements, or other treatments that regrow or repair cartilage in the human knee. I encourage you to challenge anyone who claims otherwise.

Because we lack the technology to repair or replace those surfaces without surgery, the non-operative treatments discussed in this chapter are primarily *symptomatic relief* – meaning they make the knee feel better and more functional but do not change the cartilage structure or improve the appearance of the joint surfaces.

Let's outline what is available, what works, and what does not.

Scientific Evidence

In medicine, treatment recommendations are based on opinions and evidence. The scientific evidence that supports or refutes treatments is often mixed and is constantly evolving. As an orthopedic surgeon, I put a lot of trust in the American Academy of Orthopaedic Surgeons (AAOS) and their Guidelines for the treatment of orthopedic conditions. The guidelines are developed by workgroups of smart, diverse, and invested surgeons and researchers who are committed to letting evidence guide treatment decisions.

The Treatment of Osteoarthritis of the Knee (2nd Edition) came out in 2013 and covers the most common treatments except joint replacement [1]. The American College of Rheumatology also has some guidelines that I've taken into consideration in this Chapter [2]. I've meshed my interpretation of these two guidelines with medical literature that has been published since 2013 and my own patient experiences to form opinions printed here. While science is paramount, there is still some art to medicine. Every surgeon's opinion and experience differ.

First-Line Options – These are options that either have quality scientific research behind them or, in a few cases, are backed by limited science but are used widely or trusted by most surgeons. Most healthy patients can use these but always check with your medical practitioners to be sure.

	Cautions / Risks
Education and self-management: Patients who educate themselves and take charge of their own healthcare tend to live healthier lives and have better outcomes.	*Make sure you choose reliable sources. See the Appendix for suggestions.*
Weight loss: No treatment in this book or elsewhere has the same potential to decrease knee pain, slow the progression of arthritis, and improve your overall health like weight loss. This is a STRONG recommendation for anyone with a body mass index over thirty. See "More on Weight Loss" for more information.	*Almost no risk + high reward*
Low-impact exercise: twenty to sixty minutes of low-impact, moderate intensity exercise is recommended at least three days per week. Low impact exercises are those that don't put jarring or sudden forces on the knee. **Land-based** low-impact activities include outdoor or indoor cycling, elliptical trainer, rowing, cross-country skiing, and	*Discuss with your doctor whether this is safe.*

strength-based yoga. **Water-based** (pool) low impact exercises including swimming, water aerobics, water walking, water jogging, or using water weights in the pool. You may have to work to find exercises that fit your needs.

Mental health maintenance: Mental health is linked to pain and disability. We all need to monitor our mental health. Discuss concerns with your doctor and consider an ongoing mental health maintenance program such as meditation and mindfulness exercises. See the Appendix for suggestions on books.

Almost no risk + high reward

Physical therapy (PT): Strengthening and stretching exercises are proven to decrease knee pain in the presence of arthritis. Technique is important for muscular strengthening. I recommend a coach in the form of a therapist. Even one or two visits will help guide your program.

Avoid exercises that cause pain.

Heat and cold therapy: These are time-tested albeit typically short-term pain relievers for osteoarthritis. You can see what works best for you, but I suggest heat before and ice after exercise or activity. A shower, bath, hot tub, or heating pad can be used for heat. Ice packs or a commercially available ice machine can be used for cold therapy. Twenty minutes up to three times per day is a reasonable start. See Chapter 7 for recommendations on ice machines.

Use caution when putting ice or heating pads directly on the skin.

Cortisone injections: These are also called *steroid* or *corticosteroid* injections. Cortisone a staple treatment for knee arthritis pain.

Small risk of infection, theoretical risk of cartilage toxicity that

Cautions / Risks

Most patients get some pain relief, though results vary. Relief can range from only a few days to a few months. There is surprisingly little scientific evidence behind their efficacy, but they are so commonly given that most surgeons consider them safe and effective. Avoid cortisone injections more often than every three months, and never get one within ninety days of surgery. Diabetics should be aware of a temporary spike in blood sugars from these injections.

has not been shown clinically, avoid within ninety days of knee surgery Few patients experience a "steroid flare" with an increase in pain for 1–2 days after injection.

Non-steroidal anti-inflammatory medications (NSAIDs): NSAIDs are the primary oral medication recommended for treatment of knee arthritis pain. They work by decreasing inflammation and pain in affected joints. Over the counter **ibuprofen** (Advil® or Motrin®) and **naproxen** (Aleve®) are the best options for most patients. There are prescription NSAIDs that are more potent but have additional risks. The lowest effective dose should be used, and intermittent use is preferred over daily use.

Check with your primary care doctor on these. *Use with caution if you have a history of stomach ulcers, heartburn, bleeding disorders, blood thinner use, kidney disease, high blood pressure, heart conditions, or stroke.*

Acetaminophen (Tylenol®): Acetaminophen is a safe medication effective in some patients for arthritis pain. It is generally preferred over NSAIDs if it is effective, but some patients don't see much benefit. Acetaminophen is a great option for those who can't take NSAIDs.

Do not take with alcohol or if you have a history of liver disease. Never exceed the recommended dosages.

Topical therapies: Lotions, gels, and ointments that are rubbed into the knee have shown some benefit for arthritis pain. These are typically partial and temporary pain relievers. They make the first-line list

Low risk but read instructions and warnings on the package for these.

because they are safe, cheap, and easily accessible, but be aware that studies show unimpressive results. Most are over-the-counter. **Capsaicin cream** is probably the best over-the-counter option but must be used for 1–2 weeks to see a difference. Next are **salicylate rubs** (Bengay® and Asper-creme®) and finally **counterirritants** (Icy Hot® and Biofreeze®). Prescription NSAIDs are available in topical formulations and have some scientific evidence behind their effectiveness. Discuss this with your doctor.

Cane, crutches, walker, wheelchair: Generally, patients don't want to use one of these devices unless other options have failed. If you have concerns about balance or falling, go to this as a first-line option.

Discuss how to use these devices with your medical providers.

Second-Line Options – These are options backed by lower levels of scientific evidence or have less dramatic results in decreasing knee pain. I recommend these only when first-line options are either not effective, or a patient is unwilling or unable to undergo knee replacement surgery.

Cautions / Risks

Massage therapy: Most people love a good massage. However, there is no scientific data to prove its effectiveness for knee arthritis pain beyond temporary relief. If you can afford the cost, it may be worth trying, especially if first-line options are not available or effective.

Consider cost versus benefit.

Electrotherapeutic modalities: Some research data shows that the use of electrical stimulation of muscles and nerves around

Do not do this on your own. Discuss with your therapist first.

Cautions / Risks

the knee can be a useful adjunct to physical therapy.

Hyaluronic acid injections: These are also known as viscosupplementation injections, lubrication injections, or rooster comb injections because many pharmaceutical companies make them from hyaluronic acid extracted from rooster combs. Hyaluronic acid is a substance naturally present in the knee joint that is proposed to lubricate and cushion the joint. Considerable research has gone into these injections and the sum of that research shows unimpressive results. I only recommend these for select patients with arthritis on the milder end of the spectrum. I do not recommend them for severe knee arthritis.

Not for severe arthritis; some risk of infection; some patients have increased pain for a short period after injections.

Platelet-rich plasma (PRP) injections: These injections use concentrated products derived from a patient's own blood. They are injected into the knee joint with the idea that they can reduce pain. They do not regrow cartilage or slow the process of arthritis. The scientific research is mixed but may be reasonable to consider if you have mild or moderate arthritis. Consider the cost as your insurance may not pay for this.

Not for severe arthritis; some risk of infection; some patients have increased pain for a short period after injections; weigh the cost against modest expected benefit.

Third-Line Options – These options are reserved for those with significant knee pain from arthritis who have exhausted all other options and cannot or decline to undergo knee replacement surgery.

Cautions / Risks

Knee braces: There are not too many downsides to knee braces, but research shows modest benefits. I like **knee sleeves** made of neoprene (wetsuit material) because they retain heat and provide uniform compression around the knee. **Unloader braces** are prescription braces that have some role in *varus* and *valgus* arthritis treatment, but my experience has been that less than 50 percent of those who try these braces get meaningful relief. Overall, studies do not support their use, but they might be beneficial when all other options have failed or are unavailable.

Limited effectiveness but low risk.

Duloxetine: This is a medication typically used for depression and anxiety. There is some reasonable research showing a role for chronic knee pain from arthritis. I would only recommend it if there are no other options. Your primary care provider should prescribe it.

Check with your primary care doctor.

Options I Cannot Currently Recommend – Treatments on this list have studies showing that they are not effective, have limited evidence showing they are effective, need more research, or impose unjustifiable risk or cost to patients.

High-impact exercise: While there is a debate among medical providers as to whether high-impact activities cause arthritis, we agree that people with knee arthritis or knee pain should avoid such activities. You can increase your risks of cartilage wear and worsening symptoms by engaging in high-impact exercise.

Acupuncture: Traditional Chinese medicine treatments such as acupuncture have been around for thousands of years. I like the idea and the safety profile of this treatment, but the scientific evidence for treatment of arthritis pain isn't there. The available studies show poor results.

Therapeutic ultrasound: Ultrasound is useful as an imaging technique but far less useful as a therapeutic measure for knee arthritis.

Cupping therapy: When the most decorated Olympian of all-time competed in 2016 with cupping marks all over his body, it invigorated this alternative treatment. It lacks quality scientific support for its use in knee arthritis.

Laser therapy: Laser therapy is another alternative treatment that is not ready for mainstream acceptance based on lack of quality research.

More on Weight Loss

Weight loss can be life changing for anyone who is overweight, with or without knee pain. In order to accomplish something that is life changing, you will have to make significant changes in life. "How?" you may ask. That question is the basis of a weight loss industry worth over $70 Billion in the United States alone. Studies show that **diet is far more important than exercise when it comes to losing weight**. You must commit to a diet and use exercise as an adjunct to see progress. There is no single program that works for everyone. It doesn't matter if you count calories, weigh your food, avoid carbohydrates, start a new exercise program, join a gym, buy a book, take on one of the so-called "fad" diets. Take the following steps now if you think you are overweight:

1. Calculate your body mass index (see Chapter 2)
2. Discuss options with your medical practitioners. Some diets are healthier than others.
3. Find a support group. Tell your medical providers, family, and friends what your plan is and ask them to hold you accountable. This is not easy, and you will need support.
4. Commit to a plan. Expect it to require persistent work and time. It will not be easy, but you also don't have to be perfect. You just need to make lasting changes that over time will result in weight loss.
5. **YOU** can do this!

Prolotherapy: Prolotherapy uses a sugar solution that's injected into the knee and shows promise as a future treatment option. I feel that this injection is not worth the unknown risks without more research data.

Supplements: This one is going to raise controversy and doubt. As a society, we love our supplements. Most people like the fact that they are "natural", though I would dispute this claim. If you are looking for treatments backed by science, look elsewhere. There is no supplement for osteoarthritis backed with high-quality scientific research. This includes **glucosamine** and **chondroitin**. The American Academy of Orthopaedic Surgeons states a strong recommendation against the use of either of these commonly used supplements[2]. There is a lack of scientific evidence for other commonly used supplements including: turmeric, rose hip, avocado soybean unsaponfiables (ASU), methylsulfonylmethane (MSM), willow bark, and omega-3 fatty acids. The other, potentially bigger, issue with supplements is that they are unregulated. You truly don't know what you are taking, how much you are taking, and how safe it is despite what it says on the bottle.

Shoe inserts: Insoles, orthotics, and shoe wedges all lack enough quality science showing that they reduce knee pain from arthritis.

Knee taping: Some professional athletes use and endorse kinesiology tape. That's about the best evidence I can find for its effectiveness. The science that supports taping around the knee is lacking.

Stem cell injections: I'm asked about stem cell injections at least weekly, if not daily. I have a strong recommendation against them. So far, the advertising and hype about stem cell injections for arthritis have surpassed science. There is a myriad of problems with the research, nomenclature, false advertising, and overstatement of stem cell therapeutic capabilities for arthritis. According to the American Association of Hip and Knee Surgeons (AAHKS) and the American Academy of Orthopaedic Surgeons (AAOS), "There is no data to support the idea that stem cells can sense the environment into which they are injected and repair damaged tissue [3]." Both organizations recommend against stem cell injections. The FDA has issued warnings about these injections and clinics have been fined for false advertising. Despite the great promise of stem cell treatments in medicine, knee arthritis is not ready for prime time. Do not waste your money on them until we have better research and safer formulations.

Opioid pain medications: I have an even stronger recommendation against the use of opioid medications to treat arthritis pain than for stem cell injections. Commonly prescribed opioids include oxycodone (Percocet® or Oxycontin®), hydrocodone (Norco® or Vicodin®), morphine (MS Contin®), hydromorphone (Dilaudid®), and tramadol (Ultram®). We are dealing with an opioid crisis in the United States. No country uses and abuses opiates more than we do. The AAHKS also has a position statement against opiate use for arthritis which sums up my personal opinion: "It is our position that the use of opioids for the treatment of osteoarthritis of the hip and knee should be avoided and reserved only for exceptional circumstances [4]." Don't take opioids for arthritis pain. If you are on these medications, ask your doctor to help wean you off them.

What About Knee Arthroscopy?

Many patients I see have already had the old "clean out" scope for their arthritic knee. This is occurring less frequently than in previous years because of recent research showing it has minimal benefits. There is no long-term benefit to cleaning out an arthritic knee with arthroscopy.

Remember, arthritis is a condition and not a substance. You can't just "clean out" worn cartilage and expect a good outcome. This will only expose more bone and leave behind more worn cartilage.

However, when a patient has a meniscus tear that is causing mechanical symptoms like clicking, locking, and catching, in addition to pain, a "clean out" scope may provide some relief.

Discuss this option with your surgeon. However, for most patients with advanced arthritis, I do not recommend knee arthroscopy.

What about Osteotomy?

I do not perform osteotomies. Admittedly, I have a bias against this procedure. I do not recommend it for most patients. I won't get into the details of this procedure here, but I will tell you this: only a very small subset of younger patients (typically under forty-five years old) may benefit from an osteotomy.

Osteotomies should be reserved for people with isolated *medial* or *lateral* compartment arthritis who want to remain active in impact sports. The truth is that most of these patients will eventually need a joint replacement procedure. My concern is that having an osteotomy will increase your risk of complications, including your eventual need for joint replacement.

Chapter 3 Review

- Non-operative treatments for knee arthritis cannot replace or repair cartilage.

- Try non-operative treatments before moving into knee replacement. If you find a safe and effective non-operative treatment, go with it.

- Non-operative treatments have varying degrees of scientific evidence to support their use. Rely primarily on science rather than anecdotes when choosing your treatments.

- Some of the most effective treatments are lifestyle changes: weight loss, aerobic exercise, strengthening exercises, and mental-health awareness.

- Cortisone injections, NSAIDs, acetaminophen, and topical treatments are first-line treatments. However, they have warnings.

- Consider second and third-line treatments when first-line treatments don't work or patients are not candidates for them.

- Science does not support many of the commonly used treatments for knee arthritis including acupuncture, cupping, taping, and supplements.

- Stem cell injections currently have many problems in their formulations, research, advertising, and cost. There is not enough scientific evidence to justify the risk and cost of these injections.

- Do not take opioid pain medications, except in very rare circumstances.

- Knee arthroscopy and osteotomy have limited benefits when used for knee arthritis treatment.

Chapter Four

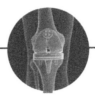

Understanding Knee Replacement Surgery

The Definitive Solution for Knee Arthritis

Your knee hurts. You've already thrown the kitchen sink of non-operative treatments at it. You might have even had a "cleanout scope". You know you need more because previous attempts to treat your knee arthritis pain have failed.

What is knee replacement and how do you know when knee replacement surgery is the next procedure to undergo? Let me arm you with more information to answer your questions.

In the previous chapter, we established that once cartilage is worn away, we do not have a reliable non-operative method to replace or repair that cartilage. The only time-tested option to replace worn cartilage is what we call a *knee replacement.*

A Brief History of Knee Replacements

The medical term for knee replacement is knee *arthroplasty*. Remember from Chapter 2 that *"arthron"* means joint. The medical term *"plasty"* means to mold or shape to restore form and function. These two words combine to form artho-plasty which is the term commonly used by medical providers. The abbreviation for *total knee arthroplasty* is TKA.

Before 1900, surgeons tried to replace worn cartilage with soft tissue structures such as tendons and fat. This method, known as *interposition arthroplasty*, was not very successful. Interposition arthroplasty continued through the early 1900s. The first time a metal piece was used to replace a portion of damaged cartilage in the knee was in the 1930s. After that, all-metal hinge-like implants followed. These ideas were innovative but had low success rates.

In 1970, unhinged devices appeared along with *polymethyl-methacrylate* bone cement which held metal and plastic pieces in place. The knee replacements took hours to perform, lasted ten years or less, and required lengthy hospital stays (several weeks or even more than a month).

Knee Replacements Today

Today knee replacements are one of the most common and most successful surgical procedures. It remains the unquestionable gold standard of treatments for severe knee arthritis (assuming patients meet other criteria discussed in Chapter 5).

More than 600,000 knee replacements are performed in the United States each year. That number is likely to double by 2030. The mean age for a knee replacement is sixty-five years; however, any adult with arthritis might qualify to have one.

Knee replacements are safely performed in small community hospitals, outpatient surgery centers, and in large medical centers. The life expectancy of a knee replacement now exceeds twenty years. The surgery typically takes 1-2 hours, and the length of stay in a medical facility ranges from hours to a few days.

What Exactly is a Total Knee Replacement?

The use of metal and plastic prosthetic pieces remains the time-tested standard used today for *total knee replacement*. The word *total* is used because it means ALL THREE compartments of the knee (Figure 4-1) are replaced at the time of surgery.

Though we call it a *total knee replacement*, the most accurate description for the modern knee replacement is a *total knee resurfacing* (nobody actually calls it this, however). The term *replacement* is common, but a bit of a misnomer because we are not replacing the entire knee joint, just resurfacing the ends of the bones.

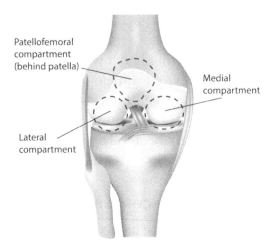

Figure 4-1: Review of the three compartments of the knee.

Let's recall what happens to the knee when cartilage surfaces are worn out. The arthritic knee has a lot of issues: worn surface cartilage, bone spurs, torn meniscus, and possibly deformity (Figure 4-2).

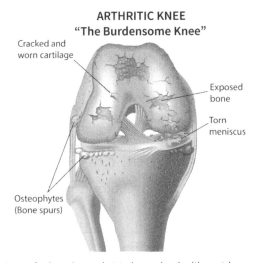

Figure 4-2: Review of what the arthritic knee looks like with worn joint surfaces.

In the United States, the most common process for resurfacing the three compartments of the knee is as follows (Figure 4-3):

1. First, the worn cartilage and soft tissues (meniscus, central ligaments, etc.) are removed from inside the joint.

2. Second, the femur, tibia, and patella are prepared to accept the new prosthetic components with a combination of special guides, drills, and saws.

3. The femur, tibia, and patella *components* (the knee replacement "parts") are attached to the prepared surfaces, usually with bone cement. The components are sized to each patient at the time of surgery and there are thousands of potential component size combinations for any given knee when you consider the four sizable parts. The femur component is always metal. There is always a plastic spacer in between the femur and tibia made of *polyethylene.* The tibia can be metal or polyethylene, and the patella is most commonly polyethylene but can be part metal and part polyethylene.

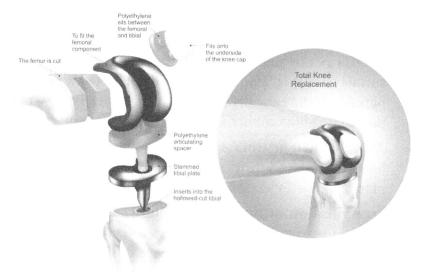

Figure 4-3: A typical knee replacement showing all of four different components. The surfaces of the femur, tibia, and patella are replaced with a combination of metal, plastic, and bone cement.

Total Knee Replacement Surgery Variables

I have just described the most common method for knee replacement in the United States. It is important to point out that there are some variables that depend purely on surgeon preference. There is a lot of debate (and no clear answer) as to whether certain variables lead to better outcomes. I suggest you go with the options that your surgeon prefers and <u>do not try to dictate these variables</u>.

For the curious patient, here is a short summary of those topics of debate. Feel free to skip this section.

- **Manufacturer/Model**: I have experience with all the major joint replacement companies for knee replacements and some of the smaller companies. I am not aware of any conclusive evidence that one brand or model is superior to others. I tell my patients that it's like asking a room full of people if Ford or Chevrolet is superior. You will get a lot of opinions, but nobody knows for sure. The implant you want is the implant your surgeon is most comfortable using.

- **Patella resurfacing**: In the United States the patella is resurfaced with a plastic or plastic/metal button more than 75 percent of the time. In Europe, this number is less than 10 percent in some countries. Both seem to work just fine.

- **All polyethylene tibia**: In some knee designs, there may not be a metal piece sitting on top of the tibia. In these cases, the plastic (polyethylene spacer) is attached directly to the tibia.

- **Free rotation of the polyethylene spacer:** Some designs have a *fixed bearing*, which means the polyethylene spacer is firmly attached to the tibia. Other designs have a *mobile bearing*, which means they allow the polyethylene spacer to rotate freely.

- **Removal of the posterior cruciate ligament (PCL):** Some knee designs remove the PCL during surgery, while others keep it.

- **Use of bone cement**: Most of the time surgeons use bone cement to attach the metal pieces to the bone. However, a growing (but small) percentage of surgeons do not use bone cement. The idea is that bone will grow into porous metal implants over time. It is not clear which method is better yet, although the use of bone cement remains the time-tested gold standard.

Partial versus Total Knee Replacement

An alternative to total knee replacement is *partial knee replacement,* which is also called a *unicompartmental knee replacement,* or simply, *uni.* A uni is offered when only one of the compartments of the knee (Figure 4-1) has significant arthritis.

Only patients with cartilage wear confined to a single compartment qualify to undergo this procedure. During a uni, the remainder of the knee outside of the arthritic compartment is left alone. An example of a partial knee replacement is shown in Figure 4-4.

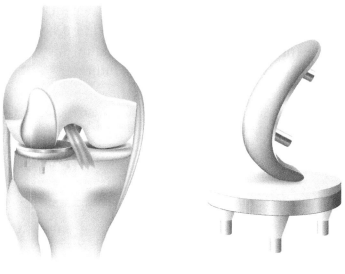

Unicompartmental
knee arthroplasty

Unicompartmental
knee implants

Figure 4-4: An example of a unicompartmental knee replacement where only the lateral compartment has been replaced.

Only your surgeon can tell you if a partial knee replacement is right for you. A unicompartmental knee replacement is an excellent procedure for the right patient. However, the "right patient" differs from surgeon to surgeon.

For me, qualifying patients must have the following characteristics:

- cartilage wear confined to one compartment
- pain centered around only that compartment
- competent knee ligaments
- a body mass index that is less than thirty-five
- good preoperative range of motion
- no inflammatory arthritis
- no excessive deformity at the knee

There are some general advantages and disadvantages of a partial knee replacement compared with a total knee replacement as shown in table 4-1. One major advantage is that most of the natural, healthy tissues are left alone. The primary disadvantage is not knowing whether the rest of the knee will or will not wear out in the future.

Table 4-1: Advantages and disadvantages of a partial knee replacement as compared with a total knee replacement

Advantages	Disadvantages
Less traumatic surgery	Uncertainty of wear in other compartments
Quicker recovery	Higher rate of long-term failure
Less intense pain with recovery	Risk of conversion to total knee replacement
More natural feeling knee (fewer clicks/clunks)	
Better short-term patient satisfaction	

Since we are not replacing the other two compartments in the knee, they are subject to wear. The ten to twenty year *survivorship* (expected lifespan) of a partial knee replacement is slightly lower than a full knee replacement. The only solution to a failed or painful partial knee replacement is to convert it to a total knee replacement. Some patients prefer a less traumatic surgery upfront and choose a uni, whereas other patients want the full knee replacement from the beginning.

Customized Knee Technology

Technology is an important part of improving outcomes in knee replacement. However, surgeons adapt technology more when clinical studies can prove that technology does one or more of the following:

- decrease complications

- increase patient satisfaction

- enhance short or long-term success rates

- aid in recovery

- decrease the overall cost of the procedure

Since each of us is unique anatomically and genetically, a customized procedure for an individual patient may lead to a better outcome. While I am convinced that we are heading toward this direction in the future, no studies have proven that customized options have a significant advantage.

Let me introduce and discuss the current customized technology for knee replacement.

- **Patient-Specific Instrumentation (PSI)**: When we cut and prepare the tibia and femur to accept metal components, the traditional method uses special jigs to make the correct angle and depth of cut. PSI utilizes a CT scan or MRI to make a 3-D model of the knee joint and customized jigs are manufactured to make those same cuts. This makes sense and sounds intriguing. Unfortunately, the literature has not shown that PSI consistently produces superior outcomes above those

of a well-trained surgeon. Some surgeons feel that this technology makes them better, and if that's the case, it's hard to
argue against. I would not request this from a surgeon that
doesn't routinely use or recommend it.

- **Custom Knee Implants:** Traditional knee replacement systems offer knee implant sizes that can fit just about any knee.
  At least one company has been very successful in marketing customizable knee implants based on a preoperative CT
  scan. The idea is more attractive to patients because they get
  a truly custom knee. However, this technology is not without issues. Sometimes, customized knee implants match the
  patient's knee before surgery but not in the operating room,
  and the surgeon may prefer a different implant size. I don't
  like the idea of being confined to a single size. Again, studies
  have not shown that these custom implants are better than
  conventional implants.

Other Knee Replacement Technology

Computer-assisted and robotic surgery have become the standard
of care in some fields of medicine. They are gaining ground in joint
replacement surgery, but like customized knee technology, studies
do not give them a significant advantage with respect to outcomes.
The downsides of other knee replacement technology are often increased costs and longer surgery times.

- **Computer-Assisted Surgical Navigation**: This technology
  uses computers and imaging to assist the surgeon in making
  bone cuts in the optimal planes. Computer-assisted surgical
  navigation is a very promising technology that will continue
  to grow, although studies do not demonstrate a significant
  advantage in terms of outcomes. Its disadvantages include
  longer surgical times and cost. I use this technology on oc-
  casion when patients have anatomic abnormalities that preclude the use of standard instrumentation, but I don't feel it
  is for every patient.

- **Robotic Surgery**: This is another area that will continue to grow. It's hard to imagine that in twenty years we will not be doing robotic and/or computer-assisted knee replacements. Today's technology has some touted advantages, but again, its outcomes are not significantly better than obtained from an experienced surgeon using standard instruments.

- **Gender-specific knees:** Patients occasionally ask if we have special knees for females. Today's joint replacement companies make products to fit almost any anatomy. One of the large joint replacement companies used to market a gender-specific knee, but it was only a marketing tool, and most companies have features available that fit female knees better, such as narrower or smaller components.

Minimally Invasive Surgery

The term *minimally invasive* refers to making a smaller skin incision and disrupting less tissue to perform a procedure. In hip replacement surgery, there have been significant advancements in minimally invasive options over the last twenty years. In knee replacement surgery, attempts to make smaller incisions have not been beneficial. In fact, some studies show worse outcomes from smaller incisions.

What most studies and surgeons agree on is that the position and size of the knee replacement components are important. In addition, the ability to account for the tightness of the surrounding soft tissue is also important. When surgeons make smaller incisions, these important factors are compromised.

Moreover, incisions have naturally gotten smaller over the years. I tell patients and surgeons that the incision should be big enough to get the job done properly. Figure 4-5 shows the typical location and size of the incision. Yours may be longer or shorter. With careful skin closure techniques, we can minimize the appearance of the incision and most patients are happy.

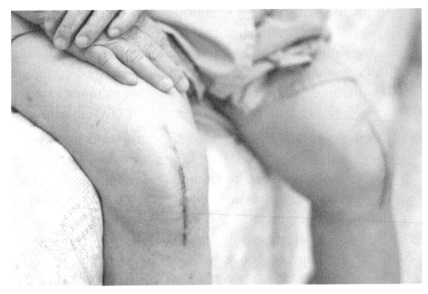

Figure 4-5: The typical location and size of a knee replacement incision. This incision is fully healed.

Same-Day Discharge Knee Replacements

Surgical equipment, surgical techniques, anesthesia techniques, medications, and other processes around knee replacement have advanced to the point where patients can go home the day of the surgery. Surgery can be performed in a stand-alone surgery center or in a hospital with same-day discharge.

Multiple studies have proven that same-day discharge is safe, and most patients are satisfied with this option. The advantages of being discharged on the same day include the comfort of staying in your own bed and having more friends and family around to help. Being at home from the beginning will also empower you to take care of yourself. One main disadvantage is that your healthcare team will not be available immediately should any complications or concerns arise.

Although same-day discharge is gaining popularity, some surgeons and hospitals won't allow it. Despite available studies, some feel it's unsafe. Other locations may not have the proper systems in place, or there may be insurance restrictions that preclude going home the same day.

The key here is that the proper systems must be in place, and patients must be properly selected for same-day discharge. It is also critical that doctors educate patients on what to expect before the surgery. Only the healthiest, most motivated, knowledgeable, and mobile patients should be offered this option.

Need Both Knees Replaced?

I often see patients who have severe arthritis in both knees and are ready to have both replaced. The question arises, how do we approach this?

Staged bilateral knee replacements is the term that describes replacing both knees on different days. The length of time between the first and second varies by patient and by surgeon. My preference is to wait a minimum of six to eight weeks before operating on the second knee – enough time to get over the initial healing phase for the first knee and prepare for the second. The overall risk of staged bilateral procedures is probably lower (some studies refute this), but patients need to plan for two big surgeries. If you choose this option, do the knee that hurts more in the first procedure, even if it has less arthritis on x-ray.

Simultaneous bilateral replacements are done on the same day, in the same surgical setting. The surgery takes roughly twice as long, and the patient takes on one recovery period instead of two. It is important to understand that this option is significantly more painful (some would say twice as painful). Some studies suggest that this option has more risks. I do not offer this option to patients unless they meet strict health criteria, and some surgeons do not do it at all because of the perceived risk.

This is a decision you should discuss with your surgeon and those caring for you. For most patients, the staged bilateral procedure is a better option.

Chapter 4 Review

- Knee replacements have evolved over the last century into one of the most successful and most common procedures performed today.

- A knee replacement replaces only the cartilage surfaces with a combination of metal, plastic, and bone cement. There are variations in technique, implants, and materials.

- Unicompartmental (partial) knee replacements are an option for select patients.

- Customized knee replacements and technology-driven options have great potential but currently show similar results when compared with traditional knee replacements.

- Minimally invasive knee replacement does not offer any benefit.

- If both knees need to be replaced, you have the choice to do them both on the same day or on two days separated by a healing period.

Chapter Five

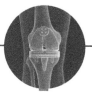

Benefits and Risks of Knee Replacement

The 85/15 Rule

Most medical treatment decisions are made based on risk versus benefit. We are constantly evaluating whether to take a pill, get an injection, or go under the knife. We often base our decisions on whether the potential benefits of these treatments or procedures justify the costs. And the costs may be in the form of money, time, or risks.

This chapter aims to help you work through the risk/benefit analysis for knee replacement. This analysis is central to determining who qualifies for the procedure.

Who Qualifies for Knee Replacement Surgery?

In my practice, patients must meet five criteria in order to move forward with a knee replacement.

1. **Moderate or severe arthritis** must be present on x-ray. Mild arthritis is not good enough to qualify a patient. In addition, MRI scans do not count for me because they often exaggerate the amount of cartilage wear.

2. **Daily, life-limiting pain symptoms** must be present. It is not worth the time, effort, and risk if the pain is mild or occasional.

3. **Non-operative measures have failed**. I want patients to have tried something else – anything else. I have a hard time jumping into surgery without at least attempting less invasive measures.

4. **Patients are healthy enough for surgery.** Most people meet this criterion, but there are some patients in which the risk of surgery exceeds the benefit. We often involve primary care providers and other medical specialists to help make this decision.

5. **Patients must understand the procedure.** By reading this book, you are covering this one. Patients and their support teams (family or friends) must understand the procedure, the risks, the benefits, and expected outcomes.

Too Young or Too Old?

Notice that age is not listed in the criteria for who qualifies for knee replacement. If you are thirty-five, have severe arthritis on x-ray, and meet the other four criteria, then it might be the right operation for you. Surgeons might hesitate with younger patients only because the patients may outlive their replaced knee, requiring a revision surgery. If you are ninety-five and meet all the criteria, then it also might be a good operation. The ninety-five-year-old must understand that medical risks of surgery are very high. The thirty-five-year-old and the ninety-five-year-old have different risk factors based on age, but they both might be good candidates for the surgery.

Benefits of Knee Replacement Surgery

Knee replacement is primarily a pain-relieving procedure. The secondary benefit is improved quality of life. Patients achieve these benefits the vast majority of the time. It is common for knee replacement patients to say after surgery, "I wish I would have done that sooner."

To say that we are aiming to decrease pain and improve quality of life is not very specific. You will notice that I did not say, "Eliminate pain and give you a perfect knee." Knee replacement is an excellent operation with very high success rates, but it's not perfect. Let us talk about what that means and how much improvement in pain and quality of life you should expect.

We cannot give you back the *invincible knee* discussed in Chapter 2. We are talking about replacing human tissue with an artificial knee made of metal, plastic, and cement. MOST patients can expect the following:

1. **Pain relief**: Most patients, though significantly improved, will not be 100 percent pain-free. Expect some minor or occasional pains even after knee replacement.

2. **Significant improvement in function**: Function has to do with how you move through each day of your life. A painful knee literally affects every step. Knee replacement should allow you to walk, put on your clothes, drive, and go to the store more comfortably and more efficiently. Note that patients with very stiff knees prior to surgery have a much higher chance of stiff knees after surgery. Stiffness is often dictated by the soft tissues around the joint. We are not replacing the soft tissues, just the joint surfaces, so this may limit the range of motion after surgery.

3. **Return to low-impact activities you previously enjoyed**: If your knee is the limiting factor for activities, replacement should help you return to those you previously enjoyed. Most patients can safely walk, hike, bike, use an elliptical trainer, swim, ski groomed runs, and play golf if they enjoyed these activities before arthritis. If other medical conditions limit these activities, the knee replacement will not overcome them.

Avoiding Misconceptions of Benefits

Let's bring some clarity to what knee replacement is NOT likely to do. The items on this list are important to understand, and most have to do with symptoms away from and not related to an arthritic knee joint.

1. **Body mass index**: Many patients believe that knee replacement will be the key to weight loss because they can exercise. It turns out that MOST patients do not lose weight after knee replacement, and some gain weight. Recall from Chapter 3 that diet is far more important than exercise for weight loss, and knee replacement does not change eating habits.

2. **Balance**: Balance worsens with age, and it is often related to systems outside of the leg and knee joint. I mention this because I have had patients who are disappointed that they still have balance difficulties after a successful knee replacement.

3. **Back pain**: It makes sense that if your gait is affected by a bad knee, the back could be affected by it. My experience has been that if your back bothers you, the knee replacement alone will not solve this problem. I suggest seeking help for both issues separately.

4. **Running, jogging, or other high-intensity sports**: Today's knee replacement is simply not made for impact activities. Activities that involve jogging, sprinting, cutting, pivoting, and jumping are not advised.

5. **Fibromyalgia or other chronic pains**: Surgery will not change any pain generated systemically outside of the knee joint.

6. **Numbness and tingling**: Numbness or tingling in your legs, feet, or toes is not likely to be caused by an arthritic knee; therefore, knee replacement will not change these symptoms.

7. **Painless clicking:** The native human knee joint has surface cartilage and meniscus that are spongy and forgiving. The replaced knee has hard surfaces made of metal and plastic. **Most replaced knees click.** This is inherent to the materials that are used, does not indicate a problem, and most patients get used to it with time.

Risks of Knee Replacement Surgery

If knee replacement surgery were always 100 percent successful, risk-free, and the replacements lasted forever, surgeons would recommend this procedure for even mild arthritis. However, every surgery carries risks. One of your surgeon's duties is to weigh your benefits against your risks.

There are three types of risks associated with a knee replacement.

1. <u>**Surgical risks**</u>: These are risks associated with the surgery itself. Luckily, complications during surgery are uncommon.

2. **Medical risks**: These are risks that happen after surgery. They are indirectly related to the surgery but caused either by the stress of surgery on the body or medications given with surgery. Medical complications occur more frequently than surgical complications.

3. **Pain and functional risks**: These risks have to do with your outcome. Even with a perfect surgery and no medical complications, pain and function after surgery can be unpredictable.

Surgical Risks

These risks are directly related to the surgery itself and/or anesthesia. During surgery, there is a small risk of bleeding, fracture of the bones, or inadvertent injury to nerves, vessels, tendons, and ligaments. Delayed surgery-related complications include infection, loosening of the prosthetic components, joint instability, and wear of prosthetic components. Anesthesia complications should also be considered but are very uncommon with modern anesthetic techniques.

I have seen many patients who cannot kneel comfortably after knee replacement. This may be a big deal for patients who kneel at their religious activities or work. Recent studies show that most patients who get knee replacements can kneel comfortably; however, just under half of them cannot kneel comfortably, making this a direct risk associated with surgery.

We lack quality studies that clearly define the percentage of patients that have surgical complications, so I'm going to give some estimates that are admittedly rough guesses based on variable scientific data. My goal is to give you an idea of the rarity of the complications above. I estimate that in the hands of an experienced surgeon, a significant complication happens during surgery less than 3 percent of the time. For example, an injury to the major artery that runs behind the knee occurs in less than 0.25 percent of patients. We have better data on delayed surgical complications. The numbers in Table 5-1 show estimates of risks based on rough averages from multiple studies.

Medical Risks

Anytime we put the human body through the stress of anesthesia and a major surgery like knee replacement, we must account for risks away from the surgery site. Not only is the surgery itself a risk, but the medications we give to help with surgery and recovery have potential side effects.

Medical complications are one of the major considerations of knee replacement surgery and depend on a patient's underlying health conditions. Examples of medical risks include blood clots in the legs or lungs or complications with the heart, lungs, liver, and kidneys. If these occur, most happen in the first few days after surgery, but the risk may extend for weeks or longer in some cases. Minor medical complications (nausea, constipation, and dizziness) are common. We are constantly watching for these and generally have answers for them. Major complications (kidney failure, heart attack, and stroke) are less common, and I estimate that significant medical complications occur less than 5 percent of the time in patients who are properly selected and medically screened before surgery.

Venous Thromboembolism (VTE)

Venous thromboembolism (VTE) is the medical term for blood clots that occur in the veins of the body. This risk deserves its own discussion because it can happen in any patient and has the potential to be serious. The two primary places blood clots occur are in the legs (called *deep vein thrombosis* or *DVT*) and in the lungs (called *pulmonary embolism* or *PE*). Treatments that attempt to avoid a complication are termed *prophylaxis*. Without VTE prophylaxis, some studies quote rates of higher than 50 percent for DVT and PE. With proper prophylaxis, that rate drops to around 1-2 percent.

We think about VTE for two reasons. First, DVT can cause a lot of pain and swelling in the legs. Secondly, if a PE forms in the lungs, it can be life-threatening. Prophylactic measures that help avoid VTE include activating your leg muscles after surgery, using special compression devices on the legs, and using a blood thinning medication.

This topic will be discussed further in Chapters 9 and 10 when we discuss recovery after surgery.

Table 5-1: Risks with knee replacements (approximate)

Risk	Approximate Incidence (varies between studies)
Unexplained pain	5–10%
Stiffness	5–7%
Loosening of components	3–5%
Symptomatic DVT or PE	1–2%
Major medical complications	<5%
Neurologic or vascular injury	<1%
Infection	1%

Pain and Functional Risks

Even when your surgery goes perfectly and there are no medical complications and even when you follow your postoperative rehabilitation instructions to the letter, there is a risk that pain and function will not meet your expectations. This is one of the most unpredictable parts of knee replacement.

Studies show that around 5 percent to 10 percent of patients will have unexplained pain or functional issues after surgery without an identifiable cause. When pain is present and there is no obvious cause, it is frustrating for the patient and the medical team.

Stiffness in the knee is also a symptom that can occur post-surgery. Any time we do surgery, the body's response is to heal with scar tissue. Scar tissue is not as stretchy and mobile as native tissues. The more stiffness you have before surgery, the greater the risk of stiffness after surgery. Physical therapy and a strict knee exercise program can help avoid this.

Successful Surgery and the 85/15 Rule

There is debate in the orthopedic community about how to gauge the success of a surgery. Do we judge it by complications, patient satisfaction with the process, or patient satisfaction with the outcome? The answers to these questions are not clear.

Researchers have developed questionnaires to determine patient satisfaction, and, in my opinion, these are the best current measure of success. If you can answer "Yes" to the question, "Are you satisfied with your knee replacement?" then it was the right decision. The answer to this question takes into account complications, pain, and function, and is different from the questions, "Is your knee perfect?" or "Did you have any complications?"

Here is where we end up with what I call "*The 85/15 Rule.*" Most studies show that patient satisfaction after knee replacement is between 80 and 90 percent. I take an average of those numbers and state that about **85 percent of patients are happy** and would do the surgery again if given the choice. The other **15 percent are not satisfied**. It turns out that who is satisfied and who is not depends heavily on patient characteristics.

Modifiable Risk Factors

We can influence patient satisfaction and outcomes after surgery by modifying factors within our control.

Let's go through the modifiable factors, one at a time:

- **Body mass index (BMI)**: An elevated BMI increases your risk of surgery complications. The higher your BMI, the more at risk you will be for infections, wound drainage, blood clots, complications during surgery, medical complications, pain levels after surgery, and dissatisfaction after surgery. One of my strongest suggestions to anyone with a BMI over thirty is this: commit to a diet-driven weight loss program. Anyone with a BMI over thirty should approach surgery cautiously. Patients with a BMI over forty should not have knee replacement until they've achieved significant weight loss.

- **Tobacco or nicotine use**: Nicotine causes constriction of blood vessels, impairs healing, and increases infection rates. In addition, smokers tend to have worse lung function and more pain after knee replacement. It does not matter if you smoke cigarettes, use a vaping device, chew tobacco, or use cigars – they all have nicotine. Tobacco has thousands of other chemicals that are harmful to overall health and healing. I recommend stopping the use of any nicotine-containing product at least six weeks before knee replacement. Use this surgery as your reason to quit.

- **Drug abuse:** Illicit drugs impair function, healing, compliance, social interactions, sleep, and many other negative aspects that affect surgical outcomes. If you are using them, do not consider surgery until you have completed a cessation program.

- **Alcohol use:** Consuming more than two alcoholic beverages per day in the month preceding surgery can increase the risks of complications. The liver is critical for healing after surgery, and alcohol impairs liver function with increased use. I suggest significantly limiting alcohol before surgery.

- **Blood sugar control:** This one is for diabetic patients. Patients with diabetes have been shown to have twice as many postoperative complications in some studies. There is a lot of debate and conflicting studies on whether *hemoglobin A1c* predicts complications after surgery. What almost everyone agrees on is that good blood sugar control before and after surgery is critical. Diabetes itself can be considered a modifiable risk factor if it's worsened by a high BMI. This is another area where a weight loss program prior to surgery is beneficial.

- **Preoperative opioid pain medications**: As recommended in Chapter 3, you should not be on opioid pain medications for arthritis pain. With an upcoming surgery, my recommendation to avoid opioids is even stronger. Studies show three important findings. First, if you are on these medications prior to surgery, pain after surgery may be more difficult to control. Secondly, patients on opioids have more medical complications after surgery and lower satisfaction rates. Finally, if you come off opioids prior to surgery, the risks mentioned reverse; meaning pain control improves, risk goes down, and satisfaction with the outcome increases.

- **Amount of knee arthritis on x-ray**: Studies have shown that patients with milder arthritis on x-ray are more likely to have pain after surgery. Nobody really knows why this occurs, but theories abound. This is why I recommend at least moderate arthritis on x-ray and prefer severe arthritis before taking on knee replacement.

- **Dentition**: Dental problems, especially when they involve cavities and infection, put patients at risk for knee joint infection after surgery. Make sure you see a dentist regularly.

- **Nutritional status**: Protein malnutrition is seen primarily in three groups: elderly, the very thin, and (paradoxically) in the obese. Nutrition is most often measured by *albumin* which is a protein measured in the blood. Several good studies have shown that low albumin levels correlate with complications.

- **Anemia:** *Anemia* is low red blood cell counts or decreased ability for red blood cells to carry oxygen via the carrier *hemoglobin*. If you have anemia going into surgery, and you lose more blood during surgery, this condition can present complications.

Non-Modifiable Risk Factors

Other risk factors are not modifiable, meaning we can't make changes to improve the risk profile.

- **Age:** We've previously established that there is no magical cutoff number that determines when a patient should and should not have a knee replacement. I find the overall health and functional status of individual patients to be more important predictors of success, so age should never be a stand-alone determinant of fitness for surgery. When we look at the population as a whole, age is a factor for complications that seems to increase more significantly after seventy-five.

- **Diabetes:** This was discussed above, and an argument can be made that diabetes is a modifiable risk factor for some patients who are obese. For others, it is not something that we can change, but it increases risks of complications, especially for patients who require insulin.

- **Heart or lung disease**: There is a very broad spectrum of severity of heart and lung disease, but your surgeon should take note of any such condition in a patient's chart to discuss the risks before surgery.

- **Liver disease:** As discussed above, the liver is a critical regulator of physiology after surgery. Patients with active liver diseases such as cirrhosis, hepatitis, or other impaired functions are at increased risk for complications.

- **Kidney disease**: Kidney function is measured by a blood test, and those with lower function are at higher risk for complications. Another concern is that patients with impaired kidney function cannot receive some of the typical medications that we give around the time of surgery.

- **Prior surgery**: Studies show that patients with any prior knee surgery have a slightly increased risk of infection with knee replacement surgery.

- **Blood disorders**: Patients who have a propensity to bleed or form clots excessively have an increased risk of complications. It is important to let your surgeon know if you have one of these disorders or take any blood thinning medications.

- **Immune deficiency:** Having an impaired immune system increases the risk of infection and decreases the body's ability to heal after surgery. Examples of diseases that can cause such impairment include HIV/AIDS and drug-induced immune deficiencies.

- **Rheumatologic disease**: Rheumatologic diseases alter the body's immune system functions, and some medications taken for these diseases do the same. Again, an impaired immune system can lead to infection and other risks.

- **Fibromyalgia or chronic pain syndrome**: These poorly understood disorders cause pain. The result after surgery is typically more pain and lower satisfaction with the result.

- **Mental health disorders**: Patients with anxiety and depression are often less satisfied with the result of knee replacement. Both disorders are linked to pain. Proper treatment can help decrease this risk.

- **Multiple medication allergies or sensitivities:** Patients with multiple reported medication allergies tend to have worse outcomes with surgery. The cause of this is not clear, but it seems that some patients are more sensitive to medications than others, and the risk of having an adverse reaction to a medication or surgery goes up when more allergies are reported. Allergies might also limit our ability to give preferred medications during and after surgery.

Chapter 5 Review

- Establishing the benefits and expectations after knee replacement is an important preoperative task. Education of patients is critical.

- Three types of risks are associated with knee replacement: surgical, medical, and pain/functional. It is important that both the patient and the medical teams understand these risks.

- Approximately 85 percent of all patients that have knee replacement are satisfied with the outcome, and 15 percent are dissatisfied. Some causes of dissatisfaction are hard to predict.

- Modifiable risk factors are those that we can change before surgery. We should make every effort to change them to maximize the outcome.

- Non-modifiable risk factors cannot be changed and understanding them is important to assess the overall risk of the procedure.

Chapter Six

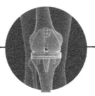

Choosing Your Team

The Right Support

Your body is like an institution. You are the CEO. If you are having a knee replacement, you have some job vacancies in your company that need to be filled. Let's discuss how to select and recruit those who are going to give you the best support and outcome.

Your Surgeon

Choosing your surgeon is not always easy. We all want the best available to do our knee replacement. There are no universal guides, formulas, or rating systems that will lead you to "the best" surgeons.

Before I go into some recommendations on how you might choose a surgeon, let me first endorse my colleagues and my profession. I am biased here, no doubt. Orthopedic surgery residencies are among the most competitive to get into out of medical school. No matter who you choose, he or she was likely at the top of their medical school class and has completed nine or more years of formal medical education and training after college. He or she has passed tests and been the subject of close scrutiny throughout their careers.

Just like any other profession, however, there is a spectrum of training, knowledge, talent, effort, and surgical skill. It is also important to point out that because of my background, training, and experience, I may value different factors when choosing a surgeon than other practitioners in this profession might value.

Choose and Trust

No single factor on the list below would cause me to rule in or rule out a surgeon from performing a quality knee replacement. Use the best information you have available to you, choose your surgeon, and, finally, trust their methods and techniques. Certainly, you should ask questions about things that don't make sense and advocate for yourself, but also trust their experience. Knee replacement surgery is a combination of science and art, and to do their best work, your surgeon needs the freedom to practice their way.

The Surgeon versus the Auto Mechanic

Orthopedic surgery has some similarities to fixing cars. Both require knowledge and manual dexterity. Both are professions where repetition and training make a difference. There are talented and knowledgeable mechanics who can fix just about anything with a combustion engine. Mechanics who are more specialized might just fix one brand or model. On average, the specialized mechanic will fix a specialized car more efficiently and accurately than the general mechanic will.

Like the auto industry, orthopedic surgery has become more sub-specialized than ever. Some general orthopedists dabble in a little bit of everything, while specialists focus on a small number of body parts. There is more to being an excellent surgeon than training, repetitions, and specialization. Innate talent, for example, is also important, and not measurable. If we are talking averages, however, it would be hard to argue against a more experienced, more specialized surgeon.

Specific Surgeon Factors to Evaluate

Each of the items listed is one part of the equation that maximizes your chances at a good outcome. None of these factors is a stand-alone dealmaker or deal-breaker when choosing your surgeon.

1. **Number of knee replacements per year**: If all else is equal, several studies have shown that the more knee replacements a

surgeon performs per year the better a patient's chance of a good outcome from a procedure performed by this surgeon. There is no well-established guideline or cutoff for the number of surgeries per year a surgeon should perform. In the absence of universally accepted definitions, I am going to give my subjective and potentially biased interpretation of the available studies. I would think twice about a surgeon who does less than thirty knee replacements per year. This is less than three per month and is *low volume*. Available studies show a clear correlation between lower volume, higher complications, and need for revision surgery. As we move closer to seventy-five knee replacements per year, my confidence starts to grow because the repetition and experience are better. Above 150 per year, a substantial portion of the surgeon's practice is dedicated to knee replacements. Most surgeons do not perform more than 300 per year, but the highest volume surgeons might do 400 or more knee replacements per year.

2. **Fellowship training**: Anyone who is licensed and credentialed to perform knee replacements in the United States has completed medical school and at least a five-year orthopedic residency training program. After residency, surgeons can go directly into practice, or they can choose to do an additional year of subspecialty training called a *fellowship*. Adult hip and knee reconstruction fellowships typically require twelve months of supervised training in primary, revision, and complex knee replacement surgeries. These are the true sub-specialists of knee replacement. The extra training is meaningful.

3. **ABOS certification**: It is surprising to some that orthopedic surgeons are not required to be board-certified to practice, though most are. The largest certifying body is the American Board of Orthopaedic Surgery (ABOS). To earn ABOS certification, surgeons must pass a written exam, be in practice for two years, and then take an oral exam. Every ten years, this certification must be updated. If your surgeon is board-certified, he or she has passed written and oral exams, and has practiced for at least two years. This combination of

experience and knowledge demonstration is helpful. For more information on board certification or to check if a potential surgeon is board-certified, the ABOS has a useful look-up site: https://mycertifiedorthopaedicsurgeon.org

4. **Years in practice:** Years in practice can function as a bell curve with respect to surgical skill. Early in their careers, surgeons have less experience but more recent training. They also tend not to have age-related physical limitations. At the back end of a surgical career, experience peaks. However, surgeons are less likely to take on new techniques very late in their careers and aging often leads to a decline in sensory and motor skills. Let us estimate that a typical surgical career is around thirty years. I've always felt that the middle twenty years of that career are probably a surgeon's best. This phase of the career balances experience, skill, drive, receptiveness to innovation, and physical dexterity.

5. **Professional reputation:** If you know someone who works in a local orthopedic clinic, hospital, or especially an operating room, this might be a good resource. Clinic staff will know if a surgeon takes responsibility for his patients. Operating room staff will have some sense of skill and efficiency. There is one word of caution here. Surgeons are often judged in the work setting by personality and temperament. On many occasions, I have met beloved, caring, and personable surgeons with comparatively weak surgical skills, and I know surgeons with disagreeable temperaments or poor interpersonal skills who are outstanding technicians.

6. **Reputation within a community:** Community reputation is worthwhile, although it is a weak indicator of a surgeon's skill. Community reputation is influenced by many factors that have nothing to do with surgery and some that do. If a surgeon is well regarded in a community, it certainly does not hurt; just be aware that it is not everything.

Surgeon Factors That Probably Don't Matter

1. **Medical school and residency institution**: I've met many doctors since I started medical school in 2001, and I have never drawn a clear correlation between the name of a school and knowledge or skill of its graduates. The same is true for residency training. Some of the more famous Ivy League schools look good on a resume, but I can show you surgeons who went to a little-known medical school whose surgical skills exceed those of Ivy Leaguers. If your surgeon went to an accredited medical school and completed an accredited orthopedic residency program, the location or name of that institution should not be used as a pro or con in surgeon choice.

2. **Position or job title:** It has been my overall experience that if a surgeon is labeled Chief, Director, Chairperson, or maintains some other title in their department or hospital, it should not play a role in choosing him or her. These job titles are certainly earned and should be respected, but the reasons they are assigned to that role may or might not have to do with surgical skill or quality of patient care.

3. **Practice type or location**: A quality knee replacement can be performed through a large academic institution, a private hospital, an HMO, or at a small community hospital. All have potential advantages and disadvantages and this factor alone should play no role in surgeon choice. The only caveat here is that volume of joint replacements at a hospital might correlate with the quality of outcomes. This is discussed further below.

4. **Use of robots, computers, or other technology**: As was discussed in Chapter 4, we are not at a point where anyone can say definitively that the use of robots, computer navigation, or other advanced technologies consistently provide better surgical outcomes. If your surgeon uses advanced technologies and feels that he or she personally can do a better job with the technology, then I am all for it. If your surgeon believes that using conventional knee instrumentation and techniques gives him or her the

best chance at a quality outcome, then it's easy to support this approach as well. These are topics that surgeons and medical studies debate heavily, but you should remove them from your decision.

Location of Surgery

The type of hospital or surgery center and geographic location are not generally predictive of outcomes. I don't make a distinction between a hospital or a stand-alone surgery center because there are advantages to both.

However, just as surgeon expertise has some correlation with volume, the same is true for the processes and procedures in a hospital or surgery center. Nurses, surgical techs, and other support staff might have more familiarity with joint replacement patients if they care for these types of patients regularly.

An argument can also be made that more personalized care occurs at a low-volume facility, but if all else is equal, studies support lower complication rates at higher volume centers.

Physical Therapist

Choosing a therapist is a difficult task. The therapist-patient relationship is important because you will spend a lot of one-on-one time with your therapist. Patients have different preferences for style. Some want to be pushed and others want gentle care. My best advice is to start with a therapist recommended by your surgeon, family member, or friend. You might even consider booking a *prehab* (therapy before surgery) appointment to start getting familiar with your therapist and make sure it's a good fit. Establishing this relationship and expectations after surgery will benefit you both.

Over the years, I have appreciated therapists who:

1. **Have experience working with knee replacement patients:** therapists are coaches and cheerleaders for your progress. You will need reassurance that you are on track and you will need a confident therapist who knows how to offer this.

2. **Outline your plan and set goals**: patients appreciate knowing what is important at each phase of recovery. Ask for an updated plan of care at each session.

3. **Understand your personal comfort zone**: the primary concern after knee replacement is stiffness. Exercises that address stiffness are not comfortable. Surgeons rely on therapists to push you, and the good ones know how to do this without compromising your trust.

4. **Are clear about expectations and goals between appointments**: most of your physical therapy will be done outside of therapy sessions. If you expect the therapist to do the work for you, your outcome will be compromised.

5. **Provide written reports for your surgeon**: it works best if you hand-carry these reports to your surgeon appointments.

Joint Replacement Coach

I strongly recommend that you identify a joint replacement coach. A coach is someone who is close enough to you to invest in your outcome; typically, a family member or close friend. A good coach will learn the educational materials with you, attend your preoperative classes and other appointments, and be there to care for you when you get home. If you are strongly contemplating surgery or already have surgery booked, now is the time to select a coach.

Unforeseeable incidents often come up that we cannot predict. When you have the support of a close companion, it is less stressful to make decisions on how to handle these unplanned events. It is also helpful to have a second set of eyes and ears because of the volume of information you receive during this journey. Every surgeon has instructions specific to their postoperative care. Medications are usually given on a schedule and it can be helpful to have someone monitoring that. Finally, when the going gets rough, and it might, you need someone to reassure you that you will get better and that your symptoms are expected.

Help at Home

The amount of help you will need at home is patient-specific. At a minimum, I suggest that someone is available full-time for the first seventy-two hours after you arrive home from the hospital or surgery center. Once you have two to three days to gauge how much help you will need, you can reassess how much he or she needs to be there. Choose someone who is close to you. This person should be able to handle bathroom and bathing duties should the need arise. Your helper can also be your coach.

Those helping at your home should also be able to help you with meals. We will discuss meals further in Chapter 7. Most patients can stand and walk around the house but standing for extended periods to prepare meals might be difficult.

Your Driver

Assign someone to drive you to the hospital or surgery center on the day of surgery, back to your home, and around town to various post-surgery appointments. We will talk more about when you will be able to drive again in Chapter 10.

Chapter 6 Review

- Choosing your support team is an important part of the surgical process.

- Choosing the best surgeon for you is challenging. Some surgeon attributes to look for include advanced training, board certification, experience, and reputation.

- Your physical therapist will be a key player on your recovery team, and you should consider a *prehab* appointment to establish expectations.

- From your pool of close family and friends, you should select a Joint Replacement Coach, those that can help at home, and a driver. These can be the same or different people.

Chapter Seven

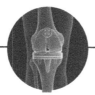

Preparing for Surgery

Set Yourself Up for Success

Knee replacement is not something you just show up and do. It takes preparation. A well-conceived preoperative plan can help set you up for a successful outcome.

Schedule Your Surgery

One of the first tasks is to schedule your surgery date. Knee replacement is elective surgery, meaning it can be scheduled well in advance and is rarely urgent. That is not to say that if the pain is severe, you should not move forward quickly. Remember from Chapter 2 that the natural history of knee arthritis is that it typically progresses slowly over time. From a technical standpoint, the surgery is usually not more difficult or risky if it is delayed a few months or even a year in most cases.

My advice is to undergo surgery when it works well with the rest of your life so give yourself time to complete the tasks in this chapter. I typically recommend a minimum of three to four weeks to complete these tasks. Coordinate the best time with your employer, your support team, and anyone else who will be affected by surgery.

Mental Preparation

Preparing mentally for surgery is a recommendation that the medical community underrates. This does not mean you should perseverate about the surgery date or stress about the outcomes. My advice is the opposite. The goals of mental preparation are to increase your awareness of how you feel emotionally and give you the mindset that maximizes your ability to deal with stress after surgery.

Stress and anxiety are very normal emotions that surround surgical procedures. It is a very different experience than what we take on in our daily lives. An important first step is to accept these emotions as normal.

If you have previously diagnosed anxiety, depression, or other mental health disorders, make sure you are happy with your current treatment plan. If you don't have a prior diagnosis but have concerns, I strongly urge you to address them with your primary care provider before surgery. Anxiety and depression are extremely common and are probably underdiagnosed. Having the awareness to address these issues is a strength and not a weakness. There are abundant resources for diagnosis and treatment.

Even if you are happy with your current mental health, I recommend mindfulness exercises as a tool, even if you are not having surgery (but especially if you are having surgery). I have no professional expertise in this field, but I've listed resources in the appendix by some who have that expertise.

Pain has cognitive, behavioral, and emotional components. The amount of pain you experience after surgery will be affected by your awareness of these components. You can start practicing some exercises before surgery that address pain. Dealing with the pain starts with an acknowledgment. I recommend very conscious and positive self-talk with phrases such as, "This hurts, but I know it will be okay," or "It's going to be difficult for a while, but I will get back on track."

Resilience plays an important role in recovering from knee replacement. I define this as the ability to adapt to stressful and painful situations and maintain a positive attitude after surgery. Resilience can improve pain levels. Research shows cognitive behavioral therapy can boost resilience after surgery, and I suggest it even for individuals with good mental health. See an introductory resource for this in the Appendix.

Physical Preparation

Ideally, patients who qualify for knee replacements would have already tried formal physical therapy to treat arthritis pain. Physical therapy is beneficial even if it does not solve the problem completely. One advantage of physical therapy is that it helps prepare your knee for surgery.

Strengthening and range of motion exercises after surgery are termed *rehab*. Exercises designed to condition the knee before surgery are called *prehab*. Performing these exercises before surgery has two main benefits.

1. It helps prepare the muscles for recovery. The stronger your muscles are before surgery, the stronger they will be post-surgery. Muscle preparation aids the recovery process.

2. It gets you in the routine of doing the same exercises you will do after surgery.

A single appointment with a licensed therapist (ideally the therapist who will help you during your postoperative rehab) is a great idea. It will give you the chance to connect with your therapist and receive advanced coaching on exercise techniques.

Similar to therapy we recommend for knee arthritis, the most important muscle groups to strengthen are the quadriceps and the hamstrings. Gentle stretching of the knee in both flexion and extension can also be helpful. As a supplemental resource, I have included some exercises in the Appendix that are effective for both prehab and rehab.

A low-impact exercise program is also important for overall health, as long as it does not cause significant pain. Do not start a new exercise routine just before the surgery. If you have time before the surgery, you will want to be in the best physical condition possible prior to it.

Eating a healthy diet is also part of your physical preparation for surgery. Do not start any new diets just before surgery but follow healthy eating guidelines. Before and after surgery it is advisable to eat a diet high in vegetables and fruit, with some protein in the form of meats, seafood, or meat substitutes.

Home Preparation

The two primary goals of preparing the home before surgery are to avoid falls and make sure the items you need are conveniently accessible. Declutter your home to avoid falls. Remove items that are a tripping or slipping hazard, including loose cords, loose rugs, toys, and small furniture. Most patients do not need to install special handrails around the house, but I recommend this if you think you might need them for an extended period after surgery.

A common question is whether you should move your bedroom to the first floor. Most patients can safely navigate a flight of stairs after surgery. You should receive instructions before discharge from the medical facility on how to go up and down stairs. If you have significant weakness or inability to go up and down stairs prior to surgery, then moving your bedroom to the first floor is not a bad idea.

Preparing or purchasing frozen meals prior to surgery is helpful. You will want quick and easy meals for the first one to two weeks. Plan a pre-surgery shopping trip to stock up, not only on food supplies but on household supplies such as toilet paper, paper towels, bathroom supplies, and other commonly used household goods.

Do your laundry just before surgery so that you have a nice stock of clean clothes. You will also want to have clean sheets on your bed when you arrive home.

Equipment to Borrow or Purchase

I recommend a four-point walker for most patients after knee replacement. The style most patients prefer is foldable (so it can fit in the car easily), has adjustable height, and has wheels on the front (Figure 7-1). While you can put your full weight on your knee after surgery, the main purpose of the walker is to improve your balance and help you avoid falls in the early recovery period. You can purchase this from a local medical supply store or online. A quality walker should cost less than $30 on amazon.com. Search for "Folding Walker with 5-Inch Wheels".

A cane is also a good idea for most patients. A few patients go directly to the cane after surgery, but most use it when they have graduated from the walker. Two styles are shown in Figure 7-1. A single-point cane is enough for most, but some prefer a four-point cane. These are available online or at drug stores for under $20.

Icing is very important after surgery. There are several options for this. The first is a commercially available ice machine. These consist of a cooler or basin filled with water and ice, tubing, and a cuff that wraps around the knee. Search "ice machine knee" on amazon. com and different styles and prices will result. Your surgeon or the hospital may also have them at a discounted price. Ice machines are not cheap, but most patients feel they are worth the cost because of the extensive amount of icing that occurs after surgery. The second option is specialized gel packs that can be frozen and wrapped around the knee. The third option is large frozen vegetable bags (peas tend to work well). Last, plastic bags filled with ice can be used. You'll want to purchase large freezer bags that seal for this.

For rehab, another optional device is a specialized pillow. I have a personal preference for one called the Knee Buddy Extender made by Bone Foam®. This device is great because it allows you to elevate your foot after surgery while keeping the knee extended. It also doubles as a knee extension tool.

There are a few other recovery aids that can be helpful for home care, including an extended shoehorn, a Sock-Aid®, and a reaching/grabbing device. On amazon.com search for "knee replacement recovery kit" and several packages with these devices will result. A shower seat stool is convenient to have. This helps you to avoid standing for prolonged periods in the shower. Some patients find a raised toilet seat with handles convenient. These are not mandatory, but standard toilets are very low to the ground and it can be difficult for some to stand independently from that position for the first few weeks after surgery. The shower seat and raised toilet seat can also be ordered online for around $30 each.

A completely optional tool to purchase or borrow is a stationary bike. If you have access to a gym that has one, then having your own is not necessary. Both recumbent and upright bicycles are helpful. In my opinion, this is the best tool for postoperative rehab after a knee replacement because it addresses both strength and range of motion. How to use the bike is described further in Chapter 10 and illustrated in the Appendix.

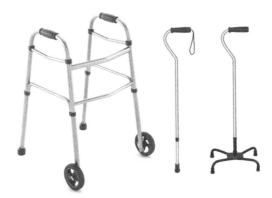

Figure 7-1: Assistive devices including a four-point wheeled walker, single-point cane, and four-point cane.

Medical Optimization

Your medical team wants you to be in the best physical condition possible for surgery. You may hear the term *medical clearance* which describes seeing a medical provider (someone other than the surgeon) prior to surgery and having that provider say that you are healthy enough to proceed. Many providers don't like the term *clearance* because it implies that surgery is either safe or not safe. As we've discussed in Chapter 5, everyone faces risks with surgery, and risks vary by patient.

You will need an appointment to evaluate your underlying medical conditions. This typically needs to be performed and documented **within thirty days of surgery.** If it is more than thirty days before surgery, you may have to repeat the exam. If you have conditions that might put you in a high-risk category for surgery, your surgeon might recommend an appointment with your primary care doctor or a specialist before the thirty-day window so that you have more time to work on medical issues.

Typical options for the optimization appointment are your primary care provider or a specialized pre-op clinic. If you don't have a primary care doctor, now is a great time to get one and have a full history and physical. A provider with expertise in medical conditions should discuss your history, perform an examination, and listen to your heart and lungs. Tests performed before surgery usually include at least an electrocardiogram (EKG) and some blood labs. Optional tests include a chest x-ray and urine sample. Depending on your history, your healthcare team may choose to order more extensive tests to examine your breathing or heart functions and check for anything that might signal a risk for surgery.

You might also employ the help of specialists. If you have a history of significant heart issues, it might be worthwhile to have a discussion with your cardiologist. If you have a neurologic disorder or have had a stroke previously, your neurologist may be helpful. The same goes for lung, kidney, liver, or any other medical issues that are chronic, for which you have seen a specialist.

In some cases, your surgeon or his or her assistant may want to meet with you just before the surgery to answer questions, discuss specifics of the surgery, sign paperwork, or accomplish some other tasks related to the surgery.

Modifiable Risk Factors and Self-Optimization

Based on your history, you may have the opportunity to improve your health prior to surgery. These topics should be discussed with your primary care doctor and your surgeon. Remember the modifiable risk factors we discussed in Chapter 5? These are so important that I'm intentionally repeating them here. You may have the option to work on them prior to surgery. In many cases, I even suggest a discussion with your surgeon on delaying surgery if you think you can make progress in any of these areas:

1. **Body mass index:** If your BMI is over thirty, I recommend weight loss. If it is over thirty-five, I strongly recommend weight loss. If it is over forty, I recommend you delay surgery until you've lost weight. Because there is a correlation between BMI and complications, you can really improve your chances of a good outcome before surgery. Make sure you lose weight in a healthy manner. It is not a good idea to do a "crash diet" right before surgery as

this might affect your nutritional status. Talk with your medical provider about the best options for you.

2. **Opioid use:** Patients who are on opioids before surgery are at risk for needing higher doses after surgery and may need more via IV. These two factors can complicate your postoperative course and increase the time you stay in the hospital. Furthermore, studies show more medical complications and higher patient dissatisfaction with surgery results when patients are on these medications before surgery. Work with your prescribing provider to decrease your use, and ideally, you should have a holiday from any opioids for one month prior to surgery.

3. **Nicotine or tobacco use:** Some joint replacement centers will no longer do elective knee replacement on patients who use nicotine or tobacco products. There is a real risk of increasing complications if you use them before or after surgery. Use surgery as a reason to quit forever. It is best to discontinue use completely at least six weeks prior to surgery. The CDC has some useful resources at www.cdc.gov/tobacco.

4. **Diabetes**: If you are diabetic, most surgeons would prefer that your hemoglobin A1c is less than eight prior to surgery. More importantly, you should closely monitor your blood sugars in the weeks leading up to surgery as well as after surgery. Check with your primary care provider if you think you need better control.

5. **Alcohol use**: I recommend you drink less than two drinks per day for a month before surgery – even better if you can abstain from alcohol. Your liver function is important for recovery, and alcohol can impede your liver.

6. **Dentist**: Make sure you don't have any cavities, infections, or other dental problems prior to surgery. If you have known problems, have them treated well before surgery. I recommend a dental appointment within six months of knee replacement. If you haven't seen a dentist in that window, make an appointment for an exam and cleaning. I recommend that you don't have any dental work done within two weeks of surgery, so plan this well ahead of time.

7.   **Sleep apnea**: Symptoms of sleep apnea include snoring, waking up a lot at night, being very tired during the day, being over-weight, or having a very large neck circumference, I suggest that you are screened for sleep apnea. Sleep apnea is a relatively common and potentially serious disorder that causes you to continuously stop and restart breathing throughout the night. This can be a dangerous disease with surgery, especially when we add medications like opioids to it. If there is any question, get it checked out prior to surgery by your primary care provider.

Metal Allergies

Since knee replacements are made of metal (most are made of cobalt-chrome), there is the risk that some patients may react to the metal. Nickel is the most commonly cited offender and there is a very small amount of nickel in cobalt chrome. Titanium is sometimes used in joint replacements as well. Both cobalt chrome and titanium are ex-tremely *inert* metals, meaning they rarely cause reactions in the body.

The subject of metal allergies is extremely complex in the knee replacement world. It is not clear whether patients who have a skin reaction or blood reaction to metals will react to orthopedic implants, and herein lies the problem with our current skin and blood testing measures. An exceedingly rare number of patients have a clinically rel-evant reaction to metals that causes pain or other problems with knee replacement surgery. You will find other surgeons and allergy special-ists who disagree with this statement. What most providers agree on is that most patients should not be screened prior to surgery. If you react to metals on the skin and you do undergo allergy testing, we don't have the answers from quality research to guide every patient in this scenario. Check with your surgeon for their preferences.

Education

By reading this book you should be getting most of the education you need before surgery. Many hospitals or surgeons offer an in-person class to help you prepare for surgery. These classes might repeat some material from this book, but also might relay information specific to your hospital or your specific surgeon. Go to this class if it is offered.

Reasons to Contact Your Surgeon Before Surgery

Even after you have set up your surgery date and followed every rec-ommendation to the letter, unexpected things may happen, and some of these occurrences may make the risk of surgery unacceptable. In these unique instances, canceling or postponing your surgery might be best for your overall health.

The list below is not all-inclusive. Some examples of when to contact your surgeon or primary care doctor immediately include:

- You become pregnant
- Infection of any type within seven days of surgery – even if you are on antibiotics
- New blood clot anywhere in the body
- New diagnosis of sleep apnea that's untreated
- New stroke or aneurysm
- New heart condition or a heart attack
- Difficulty breathing or shortness of breath
- Chest pain with exertion (example: when climbing up the stairs or exercising)
- Diarrhea or vomiting within three days of surgery
- Severe cold within three days of surgery
- New diagnosis of cancer
- You are drinking alcohol heavily or using illegal drugs
- New blood thinning medications
- You have no help at home after surgery

Chapter 7 Review

- Pick a surgery date that works for your lifestyle, family, and friends. There is no rush to undergo knee replacement.

- Preparing mentally for surgery can increase your chances of a successful outcome and decrease pain with surgery.

- Preparing physically for surgery can speed recovery. Some exercises to focus on include strength and range of motion.

- You should have a pre-operative appointment with a medical specialist prior to surgery and undergo the process of medical optimization.

- If you have modifiable risk factors for complications, you should work to minimize or eliminate these.

- Education before surgery is critical. Kudos for reading this book! If your hospital or surgeon offers a class, take it.

- There are some good reasons to delay or cancel the surgery. Contact your surgeon if you develop a new condition that might compromise your surgery results.

Chapter Eight

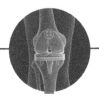

The Day of Surgery

Your Day to Relax

You read it right. Surgery day is your day to relax. For most of the knee replacement journey, it is important that you take charge and be very involved. This is the one day where you let go, put your faith in others, and go along for the ride.

If you have taken my recommendations for mental preparation, you may have some new cognitive behavioral or meditation skills to use. Regardless of your choice, try to relax and enjoy the process.

It is completely normal to be nervous. Do not apologize or worry about it. It is a natural part of this process, and there are some advantages to recognizing any anxiety and accepting it.

At Home before Surgery

The night before your surgery, try to get some good sleep. I suggest against any sleep aids unless you have cleared them with your medical providers. Avoid alcohol the night before surgery.

You should have some very clear instructions from your surgeon or the medical facility where your surgery is being performed. If you have not received these, check with your surgeon's office. These instructions might include:

- Medications to take and avoid before surgery. For example, some blood pressure medications may be taken, but some should be avoided.

- When you should have your last food or drink. This differs by facility, and there are often separate instructions for **solid foods** and **clear liquids**.

- Time of arrival for surgery. Do not be late. The operating room runs on a tight schedule and late arrival can delay other patients.

- When to shower and what type of soap to use.

- When to stop shaving your legs. Using a razor in the days leading up to surgery may increase your infection risk.

- What to wear. Dress in comfortable, loose-fitting clothes

- Don't wear makeup, perfume, cologne, aftershave, or deodorant. Some patients are very sensitive to strong scents.

- Avoid using any lotions on your skin after your last preoperative shower.

- Many centers recommend against nail polish or artificial nails because they affect the ability to read your pulse on your fingertip.

- Wear glasses rather than contact lenses.

- Remove any body piercings.

- Do not write YES, NO, or anything else on your body to indicate the correct surgery site. This causes confusion and the site will be marked by the surgical team after arrival.

- Most hospitals and surgery centers have policies against nicotine and cannabis products, and they may jeopardize your outcome, so leave them at home. If you require a nicotine patch, let your surgeon prescribe it.

Items to Bring with You

The following list consists of typical items that are recommended:

- Picture identification and insurance card
- A list of your current medications with dosages

- A credit card for co-pays
- Toiletries
- A change of clothes if you are staying overnight (loose-fitting pajamas, athletic shorts, and t-shirts are good)
- Undergarments
- Hearing aids, dentures, and eyeglasses
- A sleep apnea machine if you have one (CPAP or APAP)
- If you have a walker and cane, you might bring them so the therapists can adjust them to the proper height (ask first)
- An ice machine if you purchased one (ask first)
- Books, tablet, laptop, and/or cell phone – most hospitals have Wi-Fi available
- Flat, slip-resistant, supportive shoes

Leave these items at home unless they are specifically recommended by your surgeon or the hospital:

- Your own medications
- Cash, jewelry, and other valuables
- Contact lenses (bring eyeglasses instead)

Arrival at the Medical Facility

Aim to arrive a bit early. This can prevent anxiety and account for things such as traffic and time to walk into the surgery center. You will typically check in at a front desk. Have your photo ID and insurance card ready. You might have to pay a co-pay at this time.

The Preoperative Area

When it is your turn, you will be brought back to the preoperative area. This is where the medical team will begin to prepare you for surgery. You will probably be asked to take your clothes off and put on a hospital gown.

The nursing staff will ask you questions and make sure that you've followed your pre-hospital instructions. Answer their questions as accurately as possible. Have your medication list with dosages available. Make sure they are aware of any drug allergies. After they have completed the necessary paperwork, they will:

- Listen to your heart and lungs.

- Place an IV – this is typically in the arm or the hand.

- They may shave any hair around the incision site. It is important that you don't do this yourself before the surgery. They use a special sterile razor.

- They might wipe down your surgery site with some antibacterial wipes.

- You will likely receive some IV fluids before surgery.

- The anesthesiologist might order some pre-op medications for pain or to counteract the side effects of anesthesia.

- Some anesthesiologists will order a patch to be placed behind your ear to help with nausea.

You will meet with the anesthesiologist or nurse anesthetist prior to surgery. He or she will ask detailed questions about your medical history and your past experiences with anesthesia and will perform a brief airway exam. This is the time when the anesthesiologist has a discussion regarding what type of anesthesia to use. You should go with the recommendation. This can be a very individualized decision, and remember, he or she does this every day. You will discuss the risks and benefits of different types and will sign a form stating that you've had this discussion. There are three common options:

- **General anesthesia**: This is still commonly used and involves putting you to sleep completely. A tube is placed either down your throat or in the back of your throat to breathe for you. Some anesthesiologists prefer this on all patients, others use it for select patients.

- **Spinal anesthetic**: This is like an epidural given for childbirth, except instead of leaving a catheter in place, a single injection is given around the nerves in the lower part of your back. This removes pain sensation and renders you unable to move from the waist down. You might still feel pressure but not pain below the waist. With this option, you breathe on your own, and a sedative is also given so that you are relaxed and not aware of what is happening in the operating room.

- **Regional block**: Some anesthesiologists and surgeons prefer an injection around one of the major nerves in the hip or leg areas to cause numbness in the nerves below that location. This option is very hospital and surgeon dependent and is often given in conjunction with a general or spinal anesthetic.

Your surgeon (or possibly an assistant) will also meet with you in the preoperative area to answer any last-minute questions and have you sign the surgery consent form. The surgeon should also put his or her initials on the surgery site as a double check.

When all the preoperative tasks are complete, it's time to give hugs and kisses to loved ones and head back for surgery. You will see them before you know it with your new knee!

The Operating Room (OR)

Depending on whether you receive a sedative in pre-op, you may or may not remember much of the operating room. You will be rolled into the room on a gurney, and there will be several people present. It is normal to have one or more people from the anesthesia team, multiple surgical assistants, an operating room nurse, and possibly sales representatives that handle surgical products used by the surgeon. It is perfectly normal to be bashful about having body parts exposed that most people don't see. We have seen it all before, and we don't think twice about it. Try not to think about it and understand that these are all medical professionals who take your privacy seriously. They are there to help you and to make you comfortable.

You will be moved to an OR bed. Two devices that might be used are a urinary catheter and tourniquet. These are purely based on surgeon preference. The OR team will also get you in the correct position on the table. Don't try to help, just relax, take deep breaths, and think of your favorite place to be and who you would be with. The blood pressure cuff placed on your arm may squeeze very tightly and cause some temporary pain. This will improve. The anesthetic given through your IV may cause a significant burn in the arm. This is expected, and before you know it, the pain will go away, and you will drift off to sleep. The next thing you know, you will be in the recovery room waking up.

The process of surgery, including anesthetic, positioning, and the surgery itself, takes anywhere from one to three hours, depending on the hospital, the complexity of the surgery, and the surgeon. The time for surgery can vary, so don't let a longer or shorter-than-anticipated surgery bother you or those waiting for you.

Before you leave the operating room, a *surgical dressing* (the bandage over the incision) will be placed. Historically a drain has been placed in the knee at the end of the surgery, but good studies have shown that it makes no difference, so I find that most surgeons are not using them. The surgeon will often update your family or friends immediately following the procedure.

The Recovery Room

After the general anesthetic or sedatives have worn off, you will wake up in the recovery room. You will have a new team caring for you consisting mostly of nurses and nursing assistants. They are experienced in watching patients wake up and guiding them through the very early phases of recovery.

Very slowly, you'll sit up, start to take in ice or fluids, and maybe move on to some very simple foods. Nausea is common, so go slow. Communicate with the recovery room staff about your pain levels as they have medications available if it's not controlled. Sometimes routine x-rays are taken in the recovery room as well. Sometimes the nurses will allow your loved ones to visit you in the recovery room after you wake up.

For patients having surgery in the hospital, the recovery room is often a temporary stop before transferring you to your overnight hospital room. Once you've met certain milestones with respect to alertness, pain levels, and vital signs, and your medical condition appears stable, you will be transferred to your hospital room.

For patients going home on the day of surgery, you will spend the remainder of your time in the recovery room. Typically, you will still have to meet the same criteria for discharge as are listed in the section entitled "Criteria for Discharge Home" in Chapter 9.

Pain Control Following Surgery

In the recovery room, you will be asked about your pain levels. There are no hard rules about how much pain you will have in the recovery room or beyond. It varies greatly from person to person. How much pain you have will depend on your own physiology, what medications you've received, whether you had a spinal anesthetic or regional block, and whether the surgeon injected pain medications around the surgery site.

If you received a spinal anesthetic, regional block, or medications were injected around the surgery site, you might wake up from surgery with no pain. This is normal in some patients. Other patients wake up with pain despite these measures. If you have minimal to no pain, know that with time it is likely to increase as the medication wears off, which can be anywhere from a few hours to twenty-four hours after removal of the medication.

Measuring pain is challenging because it is a very subjective sensation. One of the common methods for assessing pain is called the visual analog scale. It is a scale where we ask patients to rate pain from 0 (no pain at all) to 10 (worst pain you can imagine). I find this tool modestly helpful because a 9 out of 10 pain for one patient might be a 3 out of 10 for another. Try to give your medical team an honest assessment.

One of the most important rules of knee replacement is this: **the goal is not to have zero pain.** This goal is not realistic and can be dangerous if you plan to achieve zero pain with pain medications. **The goal is TOLERABLE pain while resting**. For most patients, this is achieving a level 4 or less out of 10 when lying in bed or sitting. Your pain is expected to increase with movement.

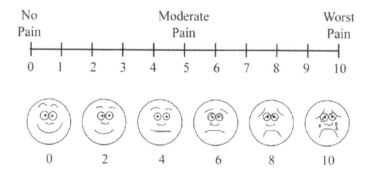

Figure 8-1: The visual analog scale used to identify pain after surgery.

Chapter 8 Review

- The day of surgery is the day you get to relax and let others work.

- Anxiety is normal on the day of surgery but do your best to relax.

- There are lists of things you should and should not bring to the hospital in this chapter that are worth reviewing before the surgery.

- Arrive early and prepare to meet several people in the preoperative area as you get prepared for the operating room.

- The anesthesiologist is your best resource to discuss anesthesia options.

- A separate team will care for you in the operating room. The surgical procedure can take anywhere from one to three hours.

- After surgery, you will spend some time in the recovery room. From there, patients who stay overnight will be moved to their overnight room.

- Pain after surgery is hard to predict. The goal for pain is never zero. Decide on what pain level is tolerable for you.

Chapter Nine

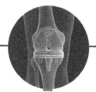

The Hospital Stay

Keep it Short

Most patients will stay at least one night in a medical facility after knee replacement. Historically, patients have stayed days or weeks in the hospital after this procedure. Over the last several years, the medical community has started to look critically at what services we are actually providing patients in the hospital, and the effect of longer stays on outcomes and complications. We have learned that as long as patients are medically stable, recovery at home is better than in a medical facility with respect to progress and outcomes. Many centers now have programs to go home on the day of surgery, which is safe for carefully selected patients. In my practice, most patients stay just one night.

Plan for the shortest stay possible. You will sleep better at home, you have more control over food and visitors, and the home provides an environment of normalcy and wellness. The sooner you get home, the faster you take control of your own recovery, which is always better than letting others wait on you.

Now, let's talk about what happens in the hospital and what it takes to get home.

The Overnight Hospital Room

From the recovery room, you will be moved to your overnight room (also called the *ward*) once some specific criteria are met. On arrival, you will meet yet another set of nursing staff that might include a nurse and nursing assistants.

Have a discussion with your nurse regarding several items to make sure you are both on the same page:

- Establish a plan and a goal for pain levels. Again, zero is not a realistic plan. Be aware that some pain medications are ordered as needed, so you will have to ask for them.

- Establish a plan for sleep. One common complaint about the hospital stay is that you are often woken up during the night to take medications or to take your vital signs. Before you go to sleep, be sure to discuss the overnight plan for these things with your nurse.

There are two common pieces of equipment used after knee replacement for blood clot prevention. The first is compression stockings. These are usually white, tight-fitting hose that go from your foot to your thigh. Whether you use them is purely surgeon preference. I have stopped using them in my practice because of the lack of scientific data showing that they prevent blood clots or swelling. Some patients find them uncomfortable. If your surgeon prefers them, I would wear them. The second item commonly used is a pneumatic compression device or *sequential compression device (SCD)*. SCDs are sleeves that utilize Velcro straps around the calves or feet. An accompanying machine injects air periodically into the sleeves so that they squeeze your legs and/or feet. This improves blood flow in the veins and decreases the risk of DVT. I use these devices for my patients. Some surgeons prescribe a mobile version to be used outside the hospital as well.

While you are in your hospital bed, I also recommend doing ankle pump exercises. These are exercises where you hold your knee straight, and alternate pointing your toes toward the ceiling and the wall in front of you (Figure 9-1). Do sets of twenty or thirty at a time with both ankles several times throughout the day. This can also keep the blood moving in the legs.

Hospital policies differ on whether family or friends can stay overnight with you. If this is allowed, it is purely your choice. The hospital will have staff available to care for you.

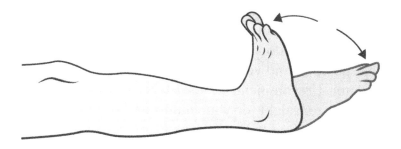

Figure 9-1: Ankle pumps - do these when resting.

Fall Risk After Surgery

Anyone who has had anesthesia and knee surgery is at risk for falls. A fall after knee replacement can be devastating, but it can be avoided with proper precautions. Never try to stand or walk without the assistance of a trained professional, especially in the first one to two days after surgery.

Early Recovery Rules

There are some important rules to follow in early recovery. These start on the day of surgery and extend for several weeks after you are home:

1. **Ice**: It is hard to use too much ice, especially during the first two weeks. This can be bags of ice, an ice gel wrap, or an ice machine (as discussed in Chapter 7). If you use ice bags or a frozen gel wrap, make sure it's not in direct contact with the skin or it may burn the skin. If you've purchased an ice machine, ask if the hospital will allow you to use it during your stay. Don't go crazy about timing ice on and off the knee, just keep it on most of the time when you are resting and take periodic breaks.

2. **Elevation**: Your knee and leg will be swollen from surgery. This happens 100 percent of the time. There is no way to eliminate it. The best way to reduce swelling is with elevation. When you are in bed, on the couch, or sitting in a chair, a good rule of thumb is "toes above the nose." The truth is that your foot should be

above your heart. Figure 9-3 shows the correct elevation of the foot. Never put a pillow under the knee and not the foot. This may be more comfortable, but you risk the knee scarring down in that position and you may have difficulty straightening your knee later. I recommend at least three pillows under the foot with the leg straight, or you could purchase the commercially available Knee Buddy Extender that I recommended in Chapter 7. This supports both the knee and the foot, elevates to the right height, and keeps the knee straight.

3. **Active versus Passive Recovery**: Knee replacement recovery is an *active recovery.* This means that you should take charge of moving around and doing your exercises. *Passive recovery* is where you lie in bed all day and have others wait on you and motivate you. One of the best ways to avoid complications is to be up on your feet, using the muscles in your legs. To start, you should be on your feet a minimum of three times per day, and the duration and frequency of this should increase with time. Never attempt to walk on your own – ALWAYS ask for assistance from the nurse.

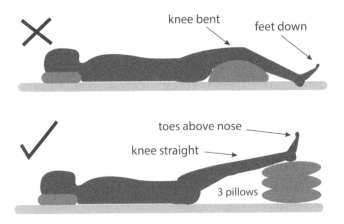

Figure 9-3: Incorrect versus correct elevation of the feet. Keep the knee straight and toes above the nose. The non-operative leg (not shown) can be in any comfortable position.

In-Hospital Therapy

The American Academy of Orthopaedic Surgeons strongly recommends starting physical therapy on the day of surgery. This seems to reduce the length of the hospital stay. I recommend that if therapy does not start, you at least get up and walk a short distance with a nurse. Do not attempt this on your own because you are at high risk for falling after surgery and anesthesia.

The physical therapists will see you once or twice per day after the first day, depending on hospital policies. Most of the time your surgeon will allow full weight on the leg after surgery and freedom to bend it as pain allows. The goal of hospital physical therapy is to get you up and walking, show you how to use a walker or cane, teach you how to climb stairs, and teach you some basic exercises to do at home. During the early phases of recovery, range of motion is far more important than strengthening exercises.

Stairs are a concern for many patients after surgery. However, patients rarely have problems once they learn the appropriate technique. The technique involves putting most of the load on your non-operative leg and taking stairs one at a time. Which leg is loaded depends on which direction you are going. The therapists should coach you in this, but the rules are:

Going up stairs: lead with the non-operative leg
Going down stairs: lead with the operative leg

You will likely also see an *occupational therapist* (OT) during your stay. The role of the OT is to teach you how to care for yourself at home. Things like how to get dressed and tools for dressing and bathing are helpful to learn before you leave.

Continuous Passive Motion (CPM) Machines

A CPM is a machine that bends and straightens your knee for you after surgery. The leg is usually strapped into the machine with Velcro straps, and it's used periodically during the hospital stay to help avoid stiffness in the knee.

Over the last ten years, these machines have become less popular. The American Academy of Orthopaedic Surgeons published guidelines in 2015 that cite strong evidence that CPMs don't improve outcomes[5]. I no longer use them in my practice, but some surgeons still find them useful.

Case Managers

A case manager may visit you as early as the day of surgery. The case manager is there to make sure that you have a safe place to go, have transportation home, have all the equipment you need, and provide resources for any other services outside the hospital. If you require a *skilled nursing facility* (rehab center) after your hospital stay, your case manager may help you arrange that.

Medical Team

Depending on your health history and hospital policies, you may have a team of medical providers visiting you in the hospital dedicated to watching over your health issues and medications outside the surgery site. Your surgeon is still in charge of surgical issues, but a medical team may assist the surgical team in managing conditions like diabetes, heart conditions, and provide recommendations when any medical issues arise after surgery. I find their input invaluable, and always welcome their help with my patients.

Criteria for Discharge to Home

I've always felt that patients should have the same discharge criteria whether they go home on the day of surgery or they stay several nights. There are criteria that take into account physical therapy goals, medical status, and making sure that the patient and the home situation is safe. Each hospital or surgery center has its own criteria, but Table 9-1 outlines some typical criteria used to make this decision.

Table 9-1: Home Discharge Criteria

Physical therapy criteria	Walk thirty feet on level ground with a walker
	Walk up and down two to three stairs
	Demonstrate understanding of home exercises
	Perform bathroom transfers
	Stand from a supine position in bed
	Be able to dress self and perform basic activities of daily living
	Equipment is available for home: walker, shower seat, etc.
Medical criteria	Tolerate a solid food diet
	Pain reasonably controlled
	Vital signs stable
	No significant nausea or vomiting
	Patient cleared for discharge by the surgical team
	Patient cleared for discharge by the medical team (if applicable)
	Able to urinate or catheter in place*
Patient criteria	Confirm availability of full-time help at home for at least seventy-two hours
	Received education on medications and home care
	Patient has a driver/ride home
	Patient/family comfortable with discharge

* In rare cases, patients cannot urinate on their own and need to have a catheter placed, which will be removed after discharge.

Education at Hospital Discharge

Once you meet your facility's discharge criteria, you will begin the discharge process. A critical component to discharge is education. Have a friend or family member present because there will be a lot of information to absorb. Make sure that you have a very clear understanding of:

- **Your medications**: timing, dosages, which require prescriptions, which are over the counter, and when to start/stop each

- **Activity levels at home**: how much weight to put on your operative leg, range of motion restrictions, basic home therapy recommendations

- **Surgical dressing**: when/if you can shower, if it can get wet, and the plan for removal

- **Physical therapy**: what is the plan for your first appointment, will it be at home or at an outpatient center?

- **Surgeon follow-up**: know the date, time, and location

- **Contacts**: who and when to call with questions/concerns

Pain Medications after Knee Replacement

The medications you take in the hospital will be similar to those you take at home. One advantage of staying overnight is that we have the opportunity to tinker with different pain medications to find the combination that works best for you.

Pain medication options include some discussed in Chapter 3 for non-operative treatment of knee arthritis. There is one major difference between pre- and post-surgery recommendations: opioid medications are appropriate for post-surgical pain. The pain medication regimen (both type and dosing) will differ between surgeons.

Most surgeons endorse what we call *multimodal pain management*, which uses several medications that work on different pain pathways rather than big doses of single opioids. Medication types will differ between patients based on your medical conditions.

Here are the most commonly prescribed options:

- **Opioids**: Commonly prescribed opioids include oxycodone (Percocet® or Oxycontin®), hydrocodone (Norco® or Vicodin®), morphine (MS Contin®), hydromorphone (Dilaudid®), and tramadol (Ultram®).

- **NSAIDs**: Common options include prescription and non-prescription types including celecoxib (Celebrex®), meloxicam (Mobic®), ibuprofen (Advil® or Motrin), naproxen (Aleve®)
- **Acetaminophen (Tylenol®):** This can be used as an adjunct medication to those above. Never take it without discussing with your medical team because some other medications may already have acetaminophen in them.

Common Side Effects of Opioids

- Nausea: if you have consistent nausea after surgery, this is the most likely culprit
- Constipation: everyone taking them should be on laxatives and stool softeners
- Dizziness, somnolence, mental cloudiness
- Skin itching or hives
- Dry mouth
- Moodiness
- Hallucinations
- Difficulty with urination
- Respiratory depression (slowed, shallow breathing) – overdose can cause death

---

Other Common Medications after Knee Replacement

Most of the other medications given after knee replacement are to counteract either side effects of the surgery or the other medications. Commonly suggested medications include:

- **Blood-thinning agent**: This is surgeon and patient-dependent, and can be aspirin, a medication injected under the skin, or one of many other pill formulations. This usually starts on the day of surgery or the day after surgery. How long to take this medication varies by the surgeon and the patient, and ranges from two to six weeks after surgery.

- **Laxatives and Stool Softeners:** If you are on opioid pain medications, you are at high risk for constipation or a more serious problem such as bowel obstruction. There are several formulations that can be purchased over the counter, and you may need to take more than one. Ask your medical team or pharmacist what is best for you.

- **Stomach acid blockers:** If you are on an NSAID or higher doses of aspirin, stomach acid blockers may be recommended to avoid stomach irritation or even stomach ulcers. There have both over the counter and prescription options. Discuss with your medical providers first.

Where to Go After Hospital Discharge

There are generally two options for where to go after hospital discharge. The first is a rehab center, which is also called a *skilled nursing facility* or *SNF*. This is a care center where you go and stay with twenty-four-hour care available. Meals are prepared for you and you undergo daily physical therapy. The second option is your own home.

I strongly advise you to make every effort to go home. Historically, more patients have gone to a rehab center, but the current trend is moving away from this option. While the SNF might sound like a good idea, there are several clear downsides. First, studies show that patients who go to a rehab center have more complications and more hospital readmissions. Just like the hospital, the rehab center exposes you to infection, and you submit to others caring for you, which leads to passive recovery. Remember we want active recovery, not passive.

A small subset of patients with significantly impaired mobility or medical problems needs closer attention than the home environment provides. If it is truly not safe to go home but you don't need the level of medical care that a hospital provides, then a rehab center is a good choice.

Chapter 9 Review

- Plan for a short stay in the hospital.

- Your nurse on the hospital ward should always assist you in standing or walking. Discuss the plan for medications and sleep.

- Ice, elevation, and walking are all important in early recovery.

- Physical therapists, occupational therapists, a case manager, and medical hospitalists may be involved in your care.

- Specific discharge criteria must be met whether you are having surgery at a surgery center or a hospital.

- Make sure you have a clear understanding of your discharge instructions and who to call before leaving the hospital.

- Where you go after surgery depends on your medical conditions and your overall function. Aim to go home rather than a rehab center if this is safe for you.

Chapter Ten

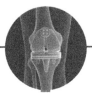

Recovery

The First 12 Weeks after Surgery

Your surgery is done, and you've got a new knee. However, the real work has just begun. I tell my patients that the surgery and the time in the hospital or surgery center are the easy part because you are guided through every step and the work is done for you. It is now your turn to put in some effort and start taking charge of your own care and your own outcome. Let us go through what to expect at each time point along the way.

Your Own Journey

This was mentioned at the beginning of Chapter 1, and it needs to be mentioned again. You will recover from knee replacement differently than anyone else. In fact, if you have both of your knees replaced at different points in time, those will be two different experiences. I strongly urge you to not compare yourself to others. You will recover more quickly/easily than some and will experience more difficulty than others. If you are concerned about progress, ask your surgeon or your therapist. They will not be bashful about telling you if you are not on track.

Pain Management at Home

Most patients need opioids for a short period of time after knee replacement. Opioids are good for short-term, post-surgical pain control if patients can handle the many side effects.

It is well published that we have an opioid epidemic in the United States. We consume 80 percent of the world's prescription opioids despite having less than 5 percent of the world population. Overdoses and visits to the emergency department are too common. The data is clear: we are overusing and abusing these drugs. Patients and doctors play a role in this. Orthopedic surgeons prescribe 8 percent of the narcotic pain medications, which puts us fourth on the list of all prescribers. No class of medications I prescribe has more side effects and complications. I am constantly examining my opioid prescribing methods and encourage that other medical providers do the same.

Opioids are terrible long-term pain relievers. Some studies estimate the addiction risk for short-term use is up to 45 percent, and if taken for more than twelve weeks, there is a 50 percent chance a patient will be using them at five years. They can change your life and your personality.

The bottom line is this: **get off opioids as soon as possible.** Transition to NSAIDs or acetaminophen as early as you can tolerate the transition. Timing is different for every patient. I have some patients who never use them after knee replacement. MOST patients can come off them after one or two weeks. I now use great scrutiny in providing them beyond four weeks and will rarely prescribe them after six weeks.

Leg Bruising and Swelling

Most patients bruise after knee replacement. Some bruise a lot. When I say a lot, I mean a continuous bruise from the thigh to the toes. Often, bruising forms around the thigh and the knee, and with time, follows gravity down toward the foot. The bruising usually starts out black, blue, or purple, and with time colors change to a lighter blue, yellow, maybe even orangish or greenish. There is nothing you can do to avoid or remove bruising other than to give it time. This is an important expectation to set: there is no amount of bruising that is concerning after knee replacement. Bruising alone never indicates a problem.

All patients have swelling after knee replacement. Some swell a lot. The location of swelling is similar to bruising – it can be anywhere from the thigh to the toes. Swelling can be a source of pain. When the skin and other soft tissues stretch from swelling, it causes a painful sensation. Swelling is something you can reduce with ice and eleva- tion. Elevation of the feet (remember, "toes above the nose") is the best way to decrease swelling.

A caveat to swelling needs to be discussed briefly. Swelling and calf pain can be signs of a blood clot in the legs (DVT). This is very difficult to diagnose and interpret because we just established that everyone has swelling in the legs, and to complicate this diagnosis further, most patients have calf pain. It is very difficult to give advice on when to seek help for this, and every surgeon has a slightly differ- ent protocol. My best advice is to discuss the protocol for diagnosing DVT with your surgeon to find out when he or she would want to be notified.

Incision, Surgical Dressing, and Bathing

Surgeons often have strict preferences on how the surgical dressing and incision are handled. Follow your surgeon's instructions closely. Some close the incision with staples and some with *sutures* (stitches). Staples need to be removed and sutures are often absorbable and do not require removal. Some surgeons use skin glue in addition to su- tures to seal and reinforce the incision. The skin glue is very much like Super Glue® but made for medical applications.

Some surgical dressings are water-resistant, while others are not. Those that are water-resistant may allow for showering but not baths, hot tubs, or swimming pools. **Check with your surgeon when showering and bathing are allowed.** To be safe you can use a combination of clear plastic kitchen wrap and medical tape to wrap in the shower (not bath) and protect it from the water. There are also some commercially available and reusable covers that you can pur- chase on amazon.com. Search "knee cast cover for shower".

The timing to remove the surgical dressing is also highly sur- geon-dependent. Some surgeons will change the surgical dressing in the hospital, and others will not. Some may have you remove it at home. Some may want to remove it in their office. Please follow their guidelines closely.

Do not let the appearance of your incision worry you in the first few weeks. The knee can be red, swollen, painful, and might even look "angry". Surgeons spend a lot of time educating patients and even other medical providers about what a normal postoperative incision looks like because it may frighten those who don't see them regularly. Be assured that the only definitive sign of early infection is persistent wound drainage, and it is rarely diagnosed in the first week after surgery. Contact your surgeon if you have any concerns.

Do not put any lotions, oils, rubs, ointments, or any other substance on your incision without clearance from your surgeon. Patients often want to get vitamin E or another substance on the scar as early as possible. There is no good evidence that these substances do anything to decrease scar appearance in early recovery, so listen to your surgeon's recommendations.

Therapy Outside the Hospital

Your therapist is an expert in exercises and recovery after knee replacement. Let him or her guide you. You should schedule your first physical therapy session before your surgery date. Aim to see a therapist within three days of your surgery. It does not matter much if you choose to have a home therapist or go to a therapy office. Although less convenient, I prefer that patients travel to the therapy office because it forces you to get dressed, get in the car, get out of the house, and walk into the therapy visit. The exercise of getting there is part of your therapy.

Your knee motion will be measured in degrees throughout your recovery. How much you can straighten the knee is called *extension*. (Figure 10-1) Full extension is designated 0 degrees. How much you can bend the knee is termed *flexion*. (Figure 10-2) Goals for flexion at different time points are discussed later in this chapter. Basic exercises to work on flexion and extension are listed in the Appendix.

The therapist is a coach and a cheerleader. He or she is there to check your progress and hold you accountable. If you rely on your therapist to do all your therapy, you will not recover well. Most of your therapy should occur on your own, at home, without the therapist present.

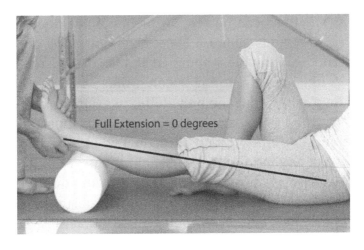

Figure 10-1: Full extension in the left knee.

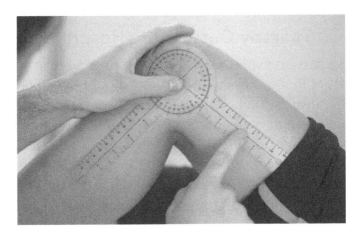

Figure 10-2: Knee flexion being measured by a therapist. This knee has about 90 degrees of flexion

The Stationary Bike

If I had to pick one recovery tool after knee replacement, it would be a stationary bike with an adjustable seat. You can use this throughout recovery for different purposes. It can help you with both range of motion and strength. It does not matter much if it's a recumbent or upright bicycle. If you don't have one, you don't necessarily need to purchase one. Most health clubs and community rec centers have several options available and purchasing a membership to one of these facilities might be advantageous as you recover and might have some benefits for your long-term health.

You should consider some instruction and supervision from a therapist. However, I have listed a stationary bike routine in the Appendix. This routine promotes extension, flexion, and strength.

Urgent Conditions

There are few concerns that come up in the first twelve weeks after knee surgery. Infection is the one we all think about, but luckily, the chance of infection is less than 1 percent.

One urgent reason to be checked out immediately is persistent blood or other fluid drainage from the knee, which may fill up the dressing. Other urgent issues are medical conditions that should concern you with or without surgery. If you have chest pain, breathing problems, or you pass out, call 911. You should be seen immediately if you have uncontrollable vomiting or diarrhea, persistent fever over 101° F, significant abdominal pain, or new/unrelenting calf pain or swelling. Your surgeon or the hospital should give you a list of reasons to call, and that list should supersede this list.

What to Expect During Weeks 0-2

Let's not sugarcoat it – the first two weeks after knee replacement are the most difficult. The level of difficulty varies from patient to patient, but this is the hardest time for most everyone. It is common for patients to wonder why they did the surgery. The good news is that if you expect and prepare for it, you will get through it just fine, and it will get better! Every day will be a step toward a better knee and life. Focus on ice, elevation, exercises, rest, and stay positive, and then repeat.

Swelling: Typically increases over the first one to two weeks.
                        Get used to it, as it will be there for several weeks.
                        Follow foot elevation and icing protocols (toes
                        above nose!)

Pain Control: Most patients will need some opioid pain medica-
                        tion and other adjunct medications. Use opioids
                        for the shortest time possible and try to discontin-
                        ue them in one to two weeks if you can.

Activity: Early on, aim to get up and walk three times per
                        day. You can start to do this at home initially. Later,
                        when you can do so comfortably and safely, you
                        can take some short walks outside. Do not overdo
                        it – you might have a setback that delays your re-
                        covery.

**Range of
motion:**   Your therapist will guide you here, but we like to
                        see you get completely straight (0 degrees) and
                        flex to 90 degrees minimum by the end of week
                        two. Many patients meet these milestones much
                        earlier than that.

**Physical
therapy:**   You should be seeing a therapist within three days
                        of surgery, and I suggest at least twice per week for
                        the first two weeks. You should be doing the ther-
                        apy exercises at least three times per day on your
                        own at home. The therapist is there to coach and
                        check your progress.

**DVT
prevention:**   Your primary blood clot prevention is movement,
                        walking, knee exercises, and ankle pump exercis-
                        es. Most patients should also be on some form of
                        medication to prevent blood clots during the first
                        two weeks after surgery.

Appointments: Most surgeons will want to see you within the first
                        two weeks after surgery. They may have an assistant
                        in their office see you on their behalf. The purpose
                        of your first appointment is to check your incision,
                        educate you, answer questions, and reassure you.

What to Expect During Weeks 2-6

You should start to see progress. Pain should start to decrease, and you should gradually increase your activity levels. You may start to enjoy the benefits of knee replacement. Remember that you are still very early in your recovery even though it may seem like you have been dealing with this knee and surgery for a while. Stay positive and do not get discouraged.

Swelling:	Should be decreasing but almost every patient still has some swelling in the knee, and possibly in the foot and ankle at six weeks after surgery.
Pain Control:	You should be off opiates as early as possible, and few patients should still be on them at four to six weeks post-surgery. If you are still on them at this point, discuss other options with your medical providers.
Activity:	Start to resume some of your daily routine. Patients often return to work and might be driving themselves around the two-to-six week range. See the discussion later in this chapter on work and driving. Walking distance varies by patient, but most should be increasing outdoor walking distance. Do not overdo it – you might have a setback that delays your recovery.
Range of motion:	Your therapist will guide you here, but we like to see you get completely straight (0 degrees) and bend to 110–120 degrees at the minimum by the end of week six. Many patients meet these milestones much earlier than that, and some will be later. Do not let it worry you if you meet the range of motion milestones later, especially if you went into surgery with a very stiff knee.
Physical therapy:	Sessions with a therapist can be dialed back if you are meeting all the milestones and are consistent about your home exercise program. Heed the advice of your therapist as to how often you should see him or her.
DVT prevention:	Your primary blood clot risk drops after two weeks, but you should still be using activity to prevent them. Depending on your surgeon's medication protocols, you may still be on a blood thinner during this time.
Appointments:	Most surgeons will want to see you in the four-to-six week range.

What to Expect During Weeks 6-12

Around weeks six to twelve, you may really start to like your knee. But will it be fully recovered? Not yet. We will discuss in Chapter 10 what full recovery looks like and how long it takes.

Most patients are very satisfied with the knee by the time they are three months out, and the good news is that it just keeps getting better after that. On average, patients are 80 percent recovered at twelve weeks, which means most of the recovery occurs in the first three months; however, there is still room for improvement.

Swelling:	Should be decreasing and minimal in most patients by twelve weeks post-op.
Pain Control:	You should be off opiates for sure, and off most of the other pain medications as well. Instead of taking scheduled doses, most patients can begin to take medications as needed.
Activity:	You should be back to your daily routine, most are back to work, most are driving, and walking longer distances outdoors should not be limited by your knee.
Range of motion:	I tell my patients that their goal is 0-120 degrees. Some will get more than this, but it is dependent on your motion before surgery and how hard you've pushed it after surgery.
Physical therapy:	Most patients complete physical therapy by six to eight weeks out from surgery, but if you and your therapist see a benefit to continuing, then I encourage that. Make sure that at your last appointment you are given a clear guideline for what you should be doing long-term to keep your knee healthy and strong.
DVT prevention:	At this point, your risk of a blood clot is close to what it was before surgery, so most patients can discontinue blood thinning medications unless your medical providers advise otherwise, or you have underlying conditions that require them.
Appointments:	Some surgeons want to see their patients at about three months out from surgery, although this is not universal.

Driving

Time to return to driving varies by patient. There are two criteria that you must meet before driving after knee surgery. First, you must be off all medications that might impede your ability to drive. This is primarily the opioid pain medications, but there might be others. Secondly, you must be able to operate the vehicle safely. This second criterion is completely up to you since your medical providers won't be able to observe you in a driving situation.

For vehicles with automatic transmission, your right foot is typically your gas-brake foot. This means that if you've had left knee surgery and are off pain medications, you may be able to drive safely. For right knee surgery or a vehicle with a manual transmission, it might take weeks to drive safely. Studies have shown that around four weeks after surgery most patients can push the brake pedal normally. Make sure you can safely do this before you get behind the wheel. Getting the blessing of your loved ones and testing your driving safety in a vacant parking lot are both advisable.

Returning to Work

Returning to work is another very individualized goal that varies greatly from patient to patient. Patients who own their own businesses or have no alternative income while they are out for surgery tend to go back earlier than those that have sick time or temporary disability policies in place. Preoperative function and postoperative pain levels also predict your return to work. Some patients start working immediately after surgery if they can work remotely and can sit for work. Some work a part-time schedule on initial return, while others wait until they can return full-time. This is your decision that you should discuss with your surgeon, your family, and your employer.

From a symptomatic standpoint, there are three things that might limit you from returning to work. The first is obvious – knee pain. The more you are on your feet doing other things, the more it is likely to swell and hurt, especially early in recovery. Secondly, knee replacement drains your energy for a few weeks. Patients report having more fatigue in early recovery than they had before surgery. Third, some jobs might not be safe to return because of physical limitations (think first-responders, laborers, need to climb ladders, etc.).

The following are averages of when patients generally return to work after knee replacement:

- Sedentary job with limited hours or remote work option: zero to four weeks

- Sedentary job, at an office location, full-time: three to eight weeks

- Non-laborer, but the job requires substantial walking/standing: six to eight weeks

- Laborer, first-responder, or need to climb ladders: eight to twelve weeks or more

Travel after Knee Replacement

For decades, orthopedic surgeons have limited travel in the initial weeks after knee replacement due to concerns for blood clots with prolonged sitting in a confined space. However, studies show that there is no significant increased risk of blood clots with post-surgery travel. You should check and see what your surgeon's recommendations are on this subject.

If you do travel, the best advice is to get up and move around frequently. Other common recommendations include the use of compression stockings, stretching your leg muscles, doing calf squeezes and ankle pumps, and staying well hydrated.

Chapter 10 Review

- Knee replacement is your own journey. Resist the temptation to compare yourself to others.

- Get off opioid pain medications as soon as you are able.

- Bruising and swelling are extremely common after knee replacement and can occur anywhere from the thigh to the foot.

- Follow your surgeon's surgical dressing, showering, and bathing recommendations closely.

- The first two weeks after surgery are the hardest, but things improve after that.

- At four to six weeks out from surgery, most people are back to their normal routine and off opioid pain medications

- By twelve weeks, your knee feels substantially better, but you are not 100 percent healed or improved or recovered yet.

- Full recovery can take six to twelve months after knee replacement.

Chapter Eleven

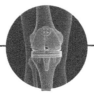

Beyond 12 Weeks

Investments and Returns

A common theme permeates throughout our human experience: the more time and effort we put into something, the more we get back from it. There are hardly any "shortcuts" or "hacks" in healthcare, and this includes knee replacement. Invest in your knee for the long term, and it will pay dividends.

What is "Full Recovery"?

Full recovery is a state of maximum improvement. This state varies for every patient. Less than 25 percent of patients will have no pain and/or symptoms. Most patients will have minimal pain complaints and/or symptoms. Patients consistently say they are satisfied and that their knees are significantly better than before surgery. If you've done your part, your strength and function will recover over time.

Most knee replacements click or have twinges of pain and mild swelling. These symptoms may not allow you to run marathons, but you may be able to do light aerobic exercise, walk, hike, bike, travel, and go to the store comfortably.

In most patients, a state of maximum improvement occurs between six and twelve months post-surgery. I've seen it take eighteen months in some patients. Time is very important in reaching this state, but you can speed it along by keeping the knee strong and staying active. This chapter is all about what you can do to get the best long-term enjoyment out of your knee.

Continuing Physical Therapy

You may be discharged from physical therapy six to eight weeks after surgery. However, your work will not be done yet. The good news is that you are guaranteed indefinite benefits when you continue to strengthen the muscles around your knee. The downside is that this requires work.

Strong muscles, particularly the quadriceps, are the key to a happy knee long-term. When you go to your last therapy appointment, talk to your therapist about what your routine should look like over the coming months. I love the stationary bike, outdoor bike, and pool as recovery tools to help you build strength and cardiovascular fitness, but you should also be doing some resistance training and weight-bearing exercises for your overall bone and joint health.

Antibiotics for Dental Visits and Other Procedures

There is much debate in the orthopedic and dental communities as to whether joint- replacement patients should take antibiotics before dental procedures. I have read through the available literature, talked to dentists as well as other surgeons, and the only thing that's clear is that there is no consensus. There are strong feelings on both sides of the subject. Everyone seems to agree that dental procedures release some normal mouth bacteria into the bloodstream. What is not clear is whether these bacteria cause artificial joint infections. The American Dental Association lists the following statement on their website:

> *In patients with prosthetic joint implants, a January 2015 ADA clinical practice guideline, based on a 2014 systematic review states, "In general, for patients with prosthetic joint implants, prophylactic antibiotics are not recommended prior to dental procedures to prevent prosthetic joint infection"[6].*

I must agree with the dentists here; the scientific studies generally show that the risk of infection of artificial joints is extremely low. Taking antibiotics may be unnecessary.

The other side of the argument is generally led by orthopedic surgeons. Most surgeons who do high-volume joint replacements have seen patients show up with joint infections shortly after a dental procedure. When this happens, the dentist usually does not hear about it and the situation can be threatening to the patient's limb. Some orthopedic surgeons' position is that a single dose of antibiotics is low risk and might prevent a disastrous infection.

My suggestion is that you talk with your surgeon and come up with a plan that you are both comfortable with.

When to See Your Surgeon

Most surgeons want patients to check in with them yearly, especially if they have enrolled you in research studies. I have found that yearly evaluation for happy patients is not necessary. If you are happy with your knee replacement, the chance of finding something abnormal that we are going to correct is very low. I think it's reasonable for happy patients to space out appointments every three to five years, but you should discuss recommendations with your surgeon.

We've established that most knee replacements are not pain and symptom-free. Most replaced knees click. Most have occasional pains and mild swelling. You should book an appointment with your surgeon if you notice a change in pain or other symptoms that don't resolve over time.

There are no sure signs of infection after knee replacement except for fluid drainage that occurs after the incision is initially healed. Fluid coming out of a previously healed incision or near a joint replacement incision is infection until proven otherwise. Contact your surgeon if you see this.

Longevity

One of the most common questions surgeons are asked is how long knee replacements last. This is a bit of a guess because we are using the best materials we have ever used, and there are many manufacturers, materials, and techniques. Based on available studies, we can expect at least 80 percent of modern knee replacements to last twenty to thirty years. Some will certainly fail before twenty years and failures are unpredictable in both cause and timing. It's rare that modern materials "wear out". Reasons for failure could be plastic wear, loosening of metal parts, infection, instability, or stiffness. Chances are that yours will last you many years, and for most patients, one knee replacement is all they will ever need.

Chapter 11 Review

- Time to full recovery varies from patient to patient, but most reach maximum improvement at six to twelve months after surgery.

- Occasional aches, pains, swelling, and clicking can be normal symptoms, especially in the first year after knee replacement.

- If you want the best possible knee function, therapy for your knee never ends. Develop a program that involves both strength and cardiovascular components to get the most out of your knee and to maximize your overall health.

- Whether to take antibiotics before dental visits is a decision you should discuss with your surgeon.

- Most knee replacements last twenty to thirty years.

Appendix

Simple Knee Motion Exercises After Surgery

Your knee range of motion (stretching) routine should be guided by your surgeon and/or therapist. In most cases, these two exercises are safe.

Knee Extension Push: Sitting on the floor or a bed, place the heel of your operative leg on a large rolled towel so that your heel is three to five inches off the ground. Use your own hands or have someone on your recovery team gently push the knee toward the ground so that it is fully straight. You will feel some discomfort. Hold for ten seconds and release. Do ten pushes, three times per day.

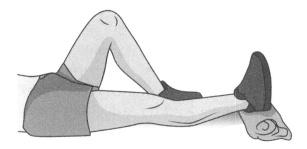

Knee Flexion Pull: Sitting on the floor or on a bed, use a small towel or your hands to pull the heel of your operative leg toward your buttocks. You will feel some discomfort. Hold for ten seconds and release. Do ten pulls, three times per day.

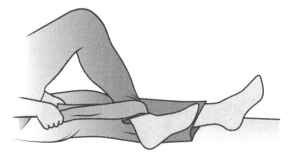

My Favorite Knee Strengthening Exercises

The quadriceps and hamstring muscle groups are the primary dynamic stabilizers of the knee joint. Some muscles around the hip also play a role in stabilizing the knee and assist with gait. The following exercises focus on strengthening these important muscle groups. The exercises shown are useful both before and after surgery. Not every exercise should be performed the day after surgery – timing is critical. I strongly recommend letting your physical therapist guide your recovery program so that each exercise is implemented at the appropriate phase of recovery.

Quadriceps Isolation: Using slow movements, move the knee through the arc of the motion shown. It is important to focus on squeezing your quadriceps muscle at the top of the arc (when the knee is fully straight). Hold the knee straight for three to five seconds, then go back down slowly. If the long arc version is painful or difficult, try one of the short arc variants. An ankle weight may be used to increase resistance. If these exercises are performed correctly, your thigh muscles should feel tired after fifteen repetitions. Aim for three sets of fifteen repetitions at least three days per week on each leg.

1. <u>Long arc quadriceps strengthening</u>: Sitting in a chair, table, or edge of an elevated bed, put the back of your knees against the edge of the sitting surface and move the knee slowly from bent to straight. Squeeze at the top!

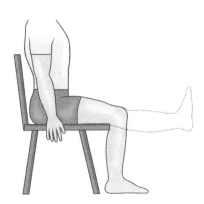

2. <u>Short arc quadriceps strengthening</u>: This is similar to the long
   arc version; however, the knee does not bend as far. Decreasing
   the bend puts less stress on your patellofemoral joint. You can
   do these in a chair or on the floor with a roll of towels under the
   knee as shown.

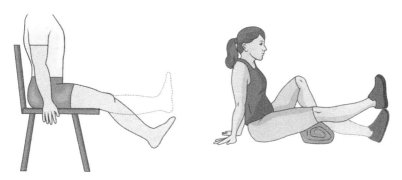

Squats: These strengthen both the quadriceps and the hamstrings.
Do whichever variant is most comfortable for you.

1. <u>Standing squat</u>: With both arms extended outward for balance,
   try to keep your back upright and bend at the knees. Go down
   only as far as you can comfortably, but do not go past a 90-degree
   bend in the knees.

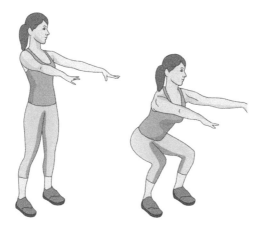

2. <u>Chair assisted squat</u>: Some people find using a chair as a reference point helpful. Try not to fully sit down on the chair. Lower and tap buttocks on it, then return to standing. Higher chars or a bed can decrease how far you need to bend your knees.

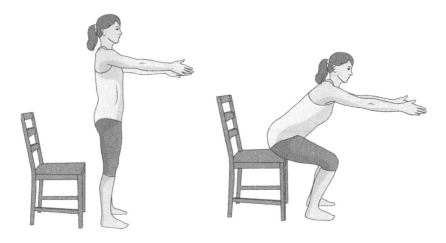

3. <u>Wall sits</u>: Using a wall for stabilization is easier for some patients than squatting up and down. Set goal times and increase as you get stronger.

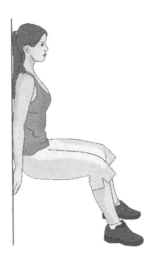

Standing Hamstring Curls: Using a chair or rail for balance, lift one foot off the ground so the knee is bent 90 degrees, hold a few seconds at the top, and return the foot to the floor. You can add ankle weights to increase resistance. Do three sets of fifteen curls for each leg at least three days per week.

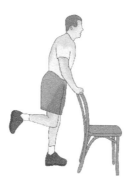

Lateral Leg Lifts: Lateral leg lifts can promote strength in some key muscles around the hip joint. Lying on your side, hold your leg straight and lift to an angle of 45-degrees with the ground, hold for two seconds, then lower your straight leg to the floor slowly. Aim for three sets of fifteen for each leg at least three days per week.

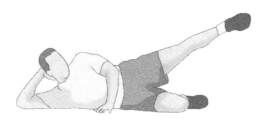

Stationary Bike: This is one of the best tools for recovering from knee surgery. It doesn't matter if you use the upright version (shown) or a recumbent bike. Riding bikes outdoors is also great, but the stationary bike provides a more controlled environment without traffic, hills, or risk of tipping over. Many patients cannot comfortably make a full revolution on the bike until two weeks post-surgery, so start by gently rocking back and forth with your feet on the pedals. It is important to check with your surgeon and your therapist to see if they have restrictions in the early recovery period. When you are cleared for the bike, I suggest the following progression of seat positions.

1. <u>High seat</u>:   Start by putting the seat at the highest level where you can still (barely) reach the pedals on both sides without your pelvis rocking back and forth on the seat. This position helps get your knee fully extended and requires the least bend to make a full revolution. Ride three to five minutes in this position making slow revolutions with minimal resistance.

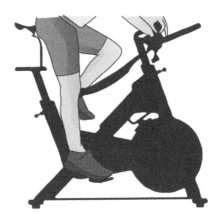

2. <u>Low seat</u>: Next, put the seat at the lowest level where you can still make a revolution with both knees. This position helps with knee flexion. Ride three to five minutes in this position with slow revolutions and minimal resistance.

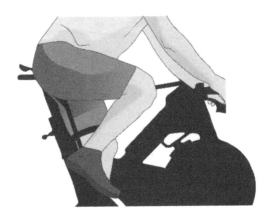

3. <u>Middle/comfortable seat</u>: The ideal seat height for normal rid-
    ing yields about a 30-degree bend in the knee when you are at
    the very bottom of the pedal stroke. With the seat in this posi-
    tion, you should be able to make a full revolution without reach-
    ing too far at the bottom or bending the knee too much at the
    top of the pedal stroke. You can turn up the resistance so that
    your thigh muscles feel fatigued. With time, increase cadence
    to ninety revolutions per minute. Work up to thirty-minute ses-
    sions with resistance, three days per week.

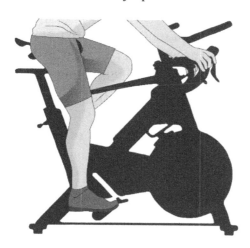

Frequently Asked Questions

Should I ask my surgeon if he or she uses recalled products? Nobody uses recalled instruments or joint replacement parts. It would be a setup for a lawsuit to knowingly use recalled products, and in the United States use of anything recalled or defective is monitored by hospitals, government agencies, companies selling the products, and the surgeons themselves. This should not be an issue.

Do I need a special card or note for airport security after knee replacement? There are no special cards or notes for airport security after knee surgery. Let TSA agents know that you have an artificial joint, and they will direct you to appropriate screening processes.

Can someone take videos or photos of my surgery? Most hospitals have policies that don't allow photos or videos in the operating room.

Can I keep any of my own bone, cartilage, or ligaments removed from the knee at the time of surgery? Most hospitals have strict policies against this, and they are typically disposed of in a sterile manner.

What is the recovery time after knee replacement? Remember, everyone is different. I tell patients it takes, on average, four to six weeks to return to most normal activities. Assume you will be close to 80 percent recovered three months after surgery. Most people require six to twelve months to reach a point of maximum improvement with respect to swelling, pain, and function.

My knee clicks or pops after knee replacement. Is this normal? Because we are replacing spongy cartilage with hard metal and plastic, some amount of painless clicking or popping is considered normal. If you are more than six months out from surgery and these clicks are associated with pain, notify your surgeon.

What about sex after knee replacement? This is a common question. Pain can limit sexual activity before and after surgery. Don't kneel on your knee until the incision is completely healed. This may take two to three months. After complete healing, let pain be your guide.

Can I go up and down stairs after total knee replacement surgery? There are typically no restrictions to stairs after knee replacement and most patients can navigate stairs within a day or two after the procedure. Discuss the technique for going up and down stairs with your therapist.

What is my range of motion goals after knee replacement surgery? The answer depends partially on your motion before surgery. In general, we aim for 0–120 degrees, which means the knee goes from fully straight (extension) to 120 degrees of bend (flexion). See Chapter 10 for more information.

Do I need antibiotics before dental work after my knee is replaced? This a controversial topic and depends on your history, your surgeon, and your dentist. See Chapter 11 for more information.

Do I need special antibiotics for other invasive procedures after total knee replacement surgery? In general, you don't need anything special, but it's always best to check with your surgeon for specific circumstances.

Do I need antibiotics when I get a cold or flu after total knee replacement surgery? Your knee replacement should not change your need for antibiotics with common illnesses. Your primary care provider should guide your use of antibiotics for cold or flu symptoms.

Is a feeling of depression normal after knee replacement? Yes! I believe this is underappreciated by patients and the medical community. The stress of surgery and the medications we typically give can make you feel tired and depressed for a period of weeks. Coming off the opiate pain medications can also cause symptoms of depression.

Is insomnia normal after knee replacement? Yes! Despite feeling tired, many patients have difficulty sleeping because of pain or medication side effects. Mindfulness exercises and a discussion with your primary care provider can help if insomnia does not improve with time.

How long will my total knee replacement last? Recent studies show that more than 80 percent of knee replacements will survive more than twenty years.

Can I get an MRI after knee replacement? Yes. The metal parts in the knee will not have any effect on the MRI in most cases. Just let the radiology team know that you have a knee replacement.

I had knee replacement three months ago and it still hurts while my friend's knee did not hurt at three months. Is this normal? There are two important points that I hope this book drills home because understanding them will affect your recovery and satisfaction. First, it takes six to twelve months for maximum improvement of symptoms, so most patients will still have pain or discomfort at three months. Secondly, everyone recovers at a different rate, so resist the temptation to compare your recovery to others.

Preoperative Checklist

- ❑ Identify your joint coach, help for home, and a driver after surgery.
- ❑ Schedule the surgery date.
- ❑ Verify with your insurance company that the surgery is covered.
- ❑ Develop a plan for mental preparation (meditation, various cognitive therapies, see a mental health provider if needed).
- ❑ Develop a plan for physical preparation (knee exercises and/or aerobic exercises).
- ❑ Develop a healthy diet plan before surgery.
- ❑ Develop a food plan for after surgery (frozen meals or have someone to cook for you).
- ❑ Search for and remove hazards for tripping, slipping, or falling in the home (rugs, cords, toys, and even small animals).
- ❑ Purchase or borrow a walker and a cane.
- ❑ Consider purchasing or borrowing optional items such as an ice machine, a knee recovery kit, and a stationary bike as outlined in Chapter 7.
- ❑ Have a plan for icing at home: ice machine, gel packs, frozen vegetables, or plastic bags with ice in them.
- ❑ Schedule your preoperative history and physical (must be within thirty days of surgery). Check with your surgeon to see if you should use a special clinic or your primary care doctor.
- ❑ Complete labs and other ordered studies well before the surgery date.
- ❑ If you smoke, stop at least six weeks prior to surgery. Use this as your reason to quit forever.
- ❑ If you are diabetic, keep blood sugars under good control leading up to surgery.

❏ Limit alcohol use to two drinks or less per day in the weeks leading up to surgery. Do not drink any alcohol for two days before your procedure.

❏ If you use opiate pain medications, stop them at least four weeks prior to surgery. Have the prescribing medical provider help you taper off them well before surgery.

❏ Schedule a joint replacement class (if one is available) or take an online course at www.OrthoSkool.com.

❏ Your surgeon, your primary care doctor, or the clinic you go to for your preoperative medical appointment should give you a list of medications to stop before surgery. Pay attention to this list as it's important.

❏ If your body mass index is more than thirty and you have time before surgery, work on weight loss. Do not go on a "crash diet" just prior to surgery.

❏ If you have not seen a dentist in the six months leading up to surgery, it's a good idea to get a checkup and cleaning. Don't have any dental work done in the two weeks prior to surgery.

❏ Make sure your vaccines are up to date well before surgery (flu, pneumonia, etc.). New flu vaccines are available in the early fall each year. Don't get any vaccinations within two weeks of your surgery date.

❏ Schedule your first post-op physical therapy appointment. Ideally, this should be within three days of the surgery date.

❏ Schedule your first postoperative appointment with your surgeon's office.

❏ Look at the list of "Items to Bring with You" in Chapter 8.

❏ Write your current medications (including dosages), supplements, and medication allergies on a piece of paper to bring with you to surgery.

❏ Put clean sheets on your bed in preparation for your arrival home.

Other Resources

Knee Arthritis

American Academy of Orthopaedic Surgeons (AAOS)
- The largest orthopedic organization in the world has an excellent patient education website that has hundreds of articles, videos, and other resources for bone and joint health: https://www.orthoinfo.org/

American Association of Hip and Knee Surgeons (AAHKS)
- You can find a lot of valuable patient information on arthritis as well as hip and knee replacements: hipknee.aahks.org
- AAHKS as some position statements on topics like stem cell therapies and opioid use here:
www.aahks.org/position-statements

American College of Rheumatology (ACR)
- A high-quality resource on various types of arthritis, particularly inflammatory conditions such as rheumatoid arthritis: www.rheumatology.org/I-Am-A/Patient-Caregiver

Mental Health and Meditation Books

10% Happier by Dan Harris, 2014.
If you are unfamiliar with meditation and mindfulness, this is an easy read and a great place to start.

The Power of Now by Eckhart Tolle, 1999.
Tolle is a visionary, teacher, and influential leader in the world of mindfulness. This book starts strong and then repeats some themes, but it has the potential to be life-changing.

Cognitive Behavioral Therapy Made Simple by Seth J. Gillihan, Ph.D., 2018.

There is some evidence that this type of therapy can help with post-operative pain. This book requires more effort than those listed above. It has strategies and exercises that may strengthen mental wellness and prepare you for surgery.

Knee Replacement Glossary

AAHKS	American Association of Hip and Knee Surgeons
AAOS	American Academy of Orthopaedic Surgeons
active recovery	Recovery from surgery that involves taking charge of your own care and moving around periodically. Contrast this with passive recovery.
albumin	A lab test that measures protein in the blood and serves as a surrogate for overall nutritional status.
anemia	Low red blood counts or low hemoglobin levels.
arthritis	An inflamed joint, usually with pain.
arthron	A Greek word meaning "joint".
arthroplasty	A term that describes reshaping a joint, or what we commonly call joint replacement.
articular cartilage	Surface cartilage in the knee joint. This covers the ends of the femur, tibia, and patella. It provides a very smooth and slick surface to facilitate joint motion with low friction.
articulate	To form a joint. To rub together.
autoimmune	A disease whereby the body produces an inflammatory reaction against normal cells.
body mass index	A formula used to assess obesity that takes into account a patient's height and weight.
bone on bone arthritis	An x-ray finding where all the cartilage space is gone on x-ray, and bones normally separated by cartilage are touching each other.
bronchitis	Inflamed bronchi (tubes in the lungs).
cartilage	A substance found in joints that serves to protect the ends of two bones forming a joint.

cartilage space narrowing	Loss of cartilage space in the knee joint, seen on x-ray or other imaging studies.
chronic	A persistent or long-term condition (versus "acute" which describes a short-term condition).
colitis	An inflamed colon.
compartments	A distinct area of cartilage within the knee. The knee has three cartilage compartments that have different wear characteristics.
components	The metal and plastic parts that we put in the knee for a knee replacement.
corticosteroid	See steroid. This is a synonym for steroid and cortisone.
cortisone	See steroid. This is a synonym for steroid and corticosteroid.
deep vein thrombosis	A blood clot that occurs in the limbs during or after surgery.
deformity	An optional feature of arthritis, whereby a joint is angulated due to underlying bone and cartilage wear.
DVT	Abbreviation for deep vein thrombosis.
dynamic	With motion. Dynamic stabilizers of the knee joint function with muscles and movement.
extension	How much your knee can straighten.
fellowship	A one-year, specialized training program that surgeons may opt to complete after residency training.
femur	The thigh bone. The longest bone in the body.
fibula	A long, thin bone in the lower leg that does not play a significant role in knee function or knee replacement surgery.
fixed-bearing	A type of knee replacement where the tibial polyethylene does not rotate.

flare	A short-term but intense increase in arthritis pain and inflammation.
flexion	How much your knee bends.
hemoglobin	The substance in red blood cells that carries oxygen. The amount of hemoglobin is measurable with a lab test.
hemoglobin A1c	A blood test used to assess sugar levels in the blood, primarily in diabetic patients.
hinge joint	A joint that bends in only one plane like a door hinge. Examples are the knee and elbow.
inert	Chemically or biologically inactive.
inflammation	The body's local response to injury or wear that is typically associated with swelling, pain, and warmth.
inflammatory arthritis	A form of arthritis where the body causes abnormal inflammation in a joint, typically due to an underlying autoimmune disorder such as rheumatoid arthritis.
inherent	Things you are born with or cannot change.
interposition arthroplasty	A historical procedure where soft tissues were used instead of metal and plastic for joint replacement procedures.
-itis	A suffix used in medicine that means "inflammation".
knee replacement	A surgical procedure where the surfaces within the knee joint are replaced with metal and plastic.
lateral	Away from the midline of the body. The lateral compartment of the knee is the one farthest away from the midline.
ligaments	Strong, fibrous, soft tissue structures that connect two bones together.
low volume	Less than thirty knee replacements per year.

medial	Toward the midline of the body. The medial compartment of the knee is the one closest to the midline.
medical clearance	A less desirable term for the medical optimization process that occurs around the time of surgery.
menisci	The plural form of meniscus.
meniscus	A c-shaped cartilage disk in the knee that helps to cushion the joint and protect the underlying articular cartilage surfaces.
mild arthritis	Mild inflammation or minimal cartilage space narrowing in a joint, usually, but not always, associated with mild symptoms.
mobile bearing	A type of knee replacement where the tibial polyethylene freely rotates on a metal tray.
moderate arthritis	A condition in between mild and severe arthritis. Typically, at least half of the cartilage space is gone on x-ray.
modifiable	Things you can change.
multifactorial	Many factors contribute to a condition.
occupational therapist	A therapist that has expertise in performing activities of daily living and self-care after surgery.
osteoarthritis	The most common form of arthritis, typically described as "wear and tear" arthritis.
osteophytes	Bone spurs.
osteoporosis	Decreased density of the bones which occurs naturally with age, more prominent in females than males.
pain	An optional feature of arthritis. Not every joint with arthritis has pain.

partial knee replacement	Only one of the three compartments in the knee is replaced and the remaining compartments are left alone.
passive recovery	Recovery from surgery that involves lying around all day and having others wait on your every need.
patella	The kneecap.
patellofemoral compartment	The compartment of the knee that includes only the patella and the trochlea.
PE	Abbreviation for pulmonary embolism.
plasty	A Greek word meaning "to mold or shape".
polyethylene	The type of plastic used in knee replacements.
polymethylmethac-rylate	The compound that makes up bone cement.
prehab	Physical therapy that occurs before a surgical procedure.
prophylaxis	A treatment given to avoid a known potential complication or disease.
pulmonary embolism	A blood clot that occurs in the lungs during or after surgery. This complication can be life-threatening.
rehab	Physical therapy that occurs after a surgical procedure or injury.
rheumatoid arthritis	The most common type of inflammatory arthritis whereby the body attacks its own cells, creating an inflammatory response and wear of cartilage.
SCD	An abbreviation for sequential compression device.
sequential com-pression device	Pneumatic compression sleeves that squeeze the legs, promoting blood flow and decreasing the risk of blood clots.

severe arthritis	Severe inflammation or severe cartilage space narrowing in a joint, usually, but not always, associated with severe symptoms.
simultaneous bilateral	A term that describes having both knees replaced in the same surgical setting, on the same day.
skilled nursing facility	Also called a SNF (pronounced "sniff"), this is a rehab center where some patients go for full-time care after surgery or an injury.
SNF	Abbreviation for skilled nursing facility.
staged bilateral	A term that describes having both knees replaced on different days. The procedures are typically separated by weeks or months.
static	Without motion. Static stabilizers of the knee joint don't require muscles to function.
steroid	A class of medications used to decrease inflammation and pain. There are oral and injectable forms. Synonyms include corticosteroid and cortisone.
surgical dressing	The bandage over the surgical incision.
survivorship	The lifespan of a knee replacement before failure or revision.
sutures	A synonym for stitches.
symptomatic relief	Addressing the symptoms of a disease without fixing the underlying problem or changing the underlying structure.
tendons	Fibrous soft tissue structures that connect muscles to bones.
tibia	The shin bone. The top of the tibia is part of the knee joint.
total knee replacement	All three compartments of the knee are replaced with metal and plastic joint surfaces.

total knee resurfacing	A more accurate description of what happens in a total knee replacement, though this term is not commonly used.
trochlea	A cartilage-covered groove in the femur where the patella slides up and down.
uni	A synonym for unicompartmental knee arthroplasty.
unicompartmental knee arthroplasty	A knee replacement procedure where only one compartment of the knee joints is replaced with metal and plastic joint surfaces.
valgus	Knock-kneed deformity in the knee joint.
varus	Bowlegged deformity in the knee joint.
venous thromboembolism	A blood clot that occurs in the veins.
VTE	Abbreviation for venous thromboembolism.
ward	An area of the hospital where patients stay overnight.

Image Credits

Selected References

1. Brown, G.A., *AAOS clinical practice guideline: treatment of osteo-arthritis of the knee: evidence-based guideline, 2nd edition.* J Am Acad Orthop Surg, 2013. 21(9): p. 577-9.

2. Hochberg, M.C., et al., *American College of Rheumatology 2012 recommendations for the use of nonpharmacologic and phar-macologic therapies in osteoarthritis of the hand, hip, and knee.* Arthritis Care Res (Hoboken), 2012. 64(4): p. 465-74.

3. *Biologics for Advanced Hip and Knee Arthritis - Position of the American Association of Hip and Knee Surgeons.* Available from: http://www.aahks.org/position-statements/biologics-for-advanced-hip-and-knee-arthritis/.

4. *Opioid Use for the Treatment of Osteoarthritis of the Hip and Knee-Position of the American Association of Hip and Knee Surgeons.* Available from: http://www.aahks. org/position-statements

5. Weber, K.L., D.S. Jevsevar, and B.J. McGrory, *AAOS Clinical Prac-tice Guideline: Surgical Management of Osteoarthritis of the Knee: Evidence-based Guideline.* J Am Acad Orthop Surg, 2016. 24(8): p. e94-6.

6. Sollecito, T.P., et al., *The use of prophylactic antibiotics prior to den-tal procedures in patients with prosthetic joints: Evidence-based clinical practice guideline for dental practitioners--a report of the American Dental Association Council on Scientific Affairs.* J Am Dent Assoc, 2015. 146(1): p. 11-16 e8.

Do you need more joint replacement education or know someone who does?

Check out these websites for an engaging, interactive, online education experience:

www.OrthoSkool.com

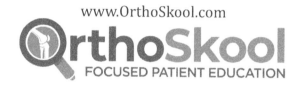

www.KneeSkool.com

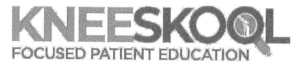

www.HipSkool.com

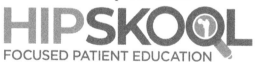

Made in the USA
Monee, IL
12 May 2024

58187340R00085